NURSING MODELS AND THE NURSING PROCESS

Nursing Models
and the Nursing Process

Peter Aggleton
Helen Chalmers

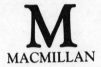

MACMILLAN

First published 1986
Reprinted 1987, 1988 (twice), 1990

Published by
MACMILLAN EDUCATION LTD
Houndmills, Basingstoke, Hampshire RG21 2XS
and London
Companies and representatives
throughout the world

Printed in Hong Kong

ISBN 0–333–41608–2 (hardcover)
ISBN 0–333–41665–1 (paperback)

The reader should note that all references in this book to
one gender should also be read as applying to the other
gender unless specifically indicated otherwise.

Contents

v

Preface

If asked, perhaps the majority of nurses today would express an interest in improving standards of care. Among them a significant proportion would probably claim that the introduction of the nursing process has been an important step towards attaining such a goal. However, as many practising nurses are only too well aware, the nursing process by itself is an essentially empty approach to care. On its own, it exhorts nurses to assess, but tells them little about *what* to assess. It encourages planning, but says little about *how* to plan. It asks nurses to intervene, but fails to say *in what ways*. It advocates evaluation, but does not specify *when* or *how*.

In the light of this, the reserve that many nurse practitioners have felt about the nursing process seems justified. In many areas of their work nurses have been expected to introduce the nursing process without a set of guidelines about how to apply it. Alternatively, the nursing process has been used uncritically to organise nursing care around a set of medical understandings of people and their needs. Both of these situations are clearly unreasonable, since they seek to deny the work of practising nurses who, over the last twenty years, have tried to develop alternative ways of thinking about people and their health-related needs. To us the use of the nursing process in this way would seem to suggest either that there is nothing that nurses can learn from each other or that they should continue to act in ways which are essentially determined by medical priorities and interests.

In producing this book our aim is to introduce practising nurses to a number of *models of nursing* which can act as guidelines for the use of the nursing process. To many nurses the idea of a nursing model may seem a strange one. Essentially, though, models of nursing are little more than sets of ideas about people and nursing care which can be used as guides for the planning and delivery of nursing care.

Contrary to the claims of writers such as Miller (1985), in writing this book we, as nurse educators, do not seek to *impose* change on nursing practice. Neither do we accept the suggestion that nurse practitioners 'rarely question the knowledge which guides their action'. We firmly believe that the relationship between nursing theory and nursing practice can only be strengthened when nurse educators turn to nurse practitioners for a critical evaluation of the ideas they propose.

Thus, within this book we aim to describe rather than criticise a number of nursing models. Our emphasis on description is a deliberate one, because it must be for practising nurses to decide on the usefulness or otherwise of nursing models. However, in the final chapter of this book we provide some guidelines about how this evaluation might take place.

In producing this book we owe a debt to friends and colleagues in Bath and Bristol, and to the many nurses we have taught since our imaginations were first aroused by the possibility of an informed yet critical nursing practice.

Bristol and Bath, 1986   P.A.
                                                                               H.C.

1

Introduction

In the last few years phrases such as 'the nursing process', 'models of nursing' and 'nursing theory' have become increasingly common in their usage. Some nurses have seen their introduction as yet another attempt to introduce jargon into practical nursing, and to make things which are simple unnecessarily complicated. Others have seen such innovations as a welcome sign that nurses are at last seeking to develop sets of understandings about people and their care-related needs distinct from those offered by the medical, natural and social sciences.

Of course, both of these positions are simplifications of what is really happening. New terminology is constantly being introduced in nursing, as it is in other walks of life. Some of the effects of this may be useful, in that they may help nurses to think about their experiences more precisely or in different ways. Others may be less so, particularly if they discourage nurses from critically thinking about the kind of care they give patients.

Likewise, the introduction of new ideas and techniques in nursing practice can lead to the development of understandings about people and their health-related needs quite different from those offered by the medical, natural or social sciences. On the other hand, it may lead us to appreciate that, in order to understand individuals and their health-related needs, the best insights from medicine, psychology and sociology should be combined with those gained from nursing practice.

The eventual outcome of attempts to develop practical nursing theory cannot be easily foreseen. In this book, therefore, a number of rather different approaches to nursing will be introduced, since this may encourage their critical evaluation. The most important task, however, will be for practising nurses to evaluate the appropriateness of each of these against the demands of their own work situations. By doing this, it may be possible to refine and develop the various approaches to nursing that follow.

Defining Some Terms

Before we look in detail at a number of approaches to planning and delivering nursing care, it would seem useful to explain certain phrases. In particular, it is important to define what is meant by the terms *the nursing process*, *nursing models* and *nursing theory*.

The Nursing Process

Until the early 1960s many nurses supposed that professional nursing practice was best achieved when based largely upon instinct and empathy. Such an approach to the planning and delivery of nursing care has tended to emphasise intuition at the expense of a more rational approach to nursing, and has since come in for considerable criticism. Bonney and Rothberg (1963) were among the first to call for a more *systematic* assessment of patients and their needs, with particular attention being paid to the physical, psychological and behavioural aspects of the individual. However, it was not until Yura and Walsh's book *The Nursing Process* (1967) that a discrete number of stages involved in nursing care came to be clearly distinguished. Yura and Walsh identified these as assessment, planning, implementation and evaluation. In arguing against a wholly intuitive approach to nursing, they advocated a more systematic and analytic approach to care. While later writers such as Little and Carnevali (1971), Mayers (1972), Crow (1977) and Marriner (1979) have spelled out in more detail what each of these stages involve, their use of the term *nursing process* seems to have certain features in common with that of Yura and Walsh. It would, therefore, seem useful to identify these.

First of all, by emphasising the value of patient *assessment*, the nursing process enables the nurse to identify with the patient

2

potential and actual problems. While some of these may have their origin within a recognised medical condition, many will be specific to individuals and to their psychological, social and cultural status. In some circumstances assessment may be a single process. More often it is divided into two stages—the first enabling a preliminary nursing diagnosis of patient problems to be made and the second facilitating an in-depth assessment, looking, in particular, for the likely causes of these problems.

Second, by arguing that nursing care should be *planned*, the nursing process encourages the nurse and the patient to set goals. These may be short-term, intermediate or long-term in nature, and specify behaviours which the patient should be able to achieve at the end of given periods of time.

Third, by identifying goals, nurses put themselves in a position to make appropriate *interventions* in order to help patients achieve them. Nursing interventions take the form of a series of activities that nurses will be involved with in order to help patients achieve goals. Some authors call these *nursing actions* (Kratz, 1979).

Finally, by emphasising the importance of *evaluation* in nursing, the nursing process encourages nurses to compare the actual behaviours patients are capable of at particular points in their care with the goals previously set. On-going evaluation of this kind is sometimes called formative evaluation, since it enables nurses to monitor the effectiveness of interventions in meeting patients'

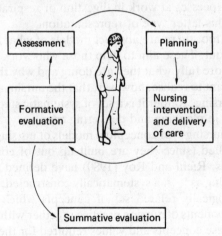

Figure 1.1   A diagrammatic representation of the nursing process

3

needs. It should not be confused with summative evaluation, which should take place after nurses have ceased to be involved in the care of particular patients.

Overall, the more questioning approach to care implied by the use of the nursing process has been an influential one in many areas of nursing since the 1960s. It would be wrong, however, to imagine that the four stages involved in the nursing process take place independently of one another. In reality, there is a continuous recycling between them as the successful completion of each step provides useful information for the next.

Nursing Models

It is important to distinguish between the nursing process—a systematic approach to care—and a *model of nursing*. In general terms, a model of something is a representation of it—a device which attempts to explain something and by so doing facilitates a better understanding of it. Some models are physical, and can be touched, manipulated, taken apart and put back together. Models of the eye and ear, of the organs within the abdominal cavity or of the brain are all examples of this type of representation. Other models are more abstract: they cannot be touched or taken apart, but they may be looked at or thought about. Diagrams showing the interrelated processes at work in digestion or respiration could be examples of this latter type of representation.

In nursing, too, there are abstract models of what nursing is, or *should be*, about. These aim to help those who work with them to understand more fully what they are doing and why they are doing it. It is important to realise, however, that the nursing process is *not* a model of nursing. Rather it is a set of systematic steps that can be gone through in planning and delivering care.

Models of nursing—or conceptual models of nursing, as they are sometimes called (since they are built up out of concepts)—are more than this. Riehl and Roy (1980) have defined a conceptual model of nursing as '. . . a systematically constructed, scientifically based, and logically related set of concepts which identify the essential components of nursing practice together with the theoretical basis of these concepts and values required for their use by the practitioner . . .'.

4

At first sight, such a definition may seem a little complicated, but careful examination reveals a number of important points which it makes about models of nursing. The most important of these is the suggestion that nursing models are *systematically* constructed. They are not simply a few bizarre thoughts and personal opinions about how nursing should take place. Instead they are developed logically, with care and effort, in an attempt to make better sense of what nurses do.

Furthermore, the development of many existing models of nursing has been influenced by research in the social and biological sciences—in particular, by discoveries in the fields of physiology, psychology and sociology. Nursing models, therefore, have not emerged out of the blue, but from a body of understanding about people and their needs often referred to as the human sciences.

However, nursing models are more than this, since they seek to use such insights to suggest practical approaches to nursing care. They do not simply take ideas from other fields of research: they actively use these to suggest better ways of nursing and caring for people. Just like their physical counterparts, models of nursing have a number of components to them. How many of these there are depends upon a model's state of development. However, either explicitly or implicitly, all of them are likely to have something to say about the aspects of patient care listed in Table 1.1.

Table 1.1   Models of nursing are likely to have something to say about the following aspects of patient care

---

(1) The nature of people
(2) The causes of problems likely to require nursing intervention
(3) The nature of the assessment process
(4) The nature of the planning and goal-setting process
(5) The focus of intervention during the implementation of the care plan
(6) The nature of the process of evaluating the quality and effects of the care given
(7) The role of the nurse

The Nature of People   Different nursing models make different assumptions about human beings and their needs. Some see people

5

as interrelated sets of anatomical parts and physiological systems. These models share some affinity with the medical model of care. Others put forward the view that it is not particularly useful to 'fragment' a person in this way, arguing instead that people are best seen as wholes, as entities more significant than the sum of their various parts. Yet other models of nursing emphasise the behavioural aspects of individuals, seeing them as people with various types of behaviour at their disposal. Others focus upon the human ability to 'philosophise' and give meaning to particular situations. Finally, there are models of nursing which try to work with several or all of these rather different approaches to understanding humans and their needs.

The Causes of Problems Likely to Require Nursing Intervention   In much the same way that models of nursing differ from one another in terms of the assumptions they make about the nature of people, they vary in terms of what they see as the likely causes of health-related problems requiring nursing intervention. Some view these in terms of anatomical or physiological malfunction. Others argue that problems arise when people are unable to adopt behaviour appropriate to the circumstances in which they find themselves. Yet others suggest that problems requiring nursing intervention arise when the overall equilibrium between people and their environment becomes disturbed.

The Nature of the Assessment Process   Models of nursing also differ in terms of how they approach nursing assessment. Some see this as a one-stage process; others see it as a series of events involving a preliminary identification of patient problems, followed by a more in-depth exploration of these. Nursing models also differ in terms of what they suggest should be attended to during the carrying out of a nursing assessment.

The Nature of the Planning and Goal-setting Process   Another way in which nursing models differ is in terms of the type of planning that they advocate nurses should carry out. Some argue that targets should be set for the return of function within anatomical parts or physiological systems. Others argue that the nurse should plan for the restoration of equilibrium within a particular aspect of a patient's behaviour. Many advocate that nurses should pay particu-

6

lar attention to the setting of goals which relate to an individual's psychological or social well-being. Most recommend that these targets be negotiated between the nurse and the patient. What all agree about, however, is that goals should be observable aspects of the patient's behaviour. It should, therefore, be apparent from what a patient says or does, when a goal has been achieved. A final contrast can be drawn between models of nursing which argue for the setting of staged goals (short-term, intermediate and long-term) and those which do not make such distinctions.

The Focus of Intervention During the Implementation of the Care Plan   By carrying out a systematic assessment of the patient and by setting realistic patient-centred goals in the light of this, the nurse will have begun to devise a plan of care. More particularly, a specific range of nursing actions or interventions is likely to be suggested by the nursing model that is being worked with, since different models of nursing suggest that different aspects of the patient should be focused on during the implementation of a nursing care plan. Some advocate holistic intervention, aiming, perhaps, to restore an overall equilibrium between individuals and their environments. Others argue that particular physiological or behavioural systems are targeted in nursing intervention. Yet others might suggest that particular attention be given to nursing actions which help to alter how people see themselves.

The Nature of the Process of Evaluating the Quality and Effects of the Care Given   Most nursing models share an overall concern that the outcomes of particular nursing interventions should be compared with goals originally set with the patient. When these seem not to have been met, the nurse is likely to want to know why this is so. Only a careful evaluation of the extent to which goals have been achieved, and the appropriateness (or otherwise) of the interventions so far used, can help to decide whether the approach to care employed has been appropriate.

Formative evaluation of this kind is central to all nursing models. However, different models vary in terms of the changes in patient behaviour to be looked for. Once again, some models of nursing emphasise changes in anatomical or physiological function. Others recommend that particular attention be given to changes in psychological status. Yet others advocate an exploration of the extent to which the person has been enabled to undertake self-care as a result of nursing intervention.

Formative evaluation of this kind, however, should not be confused with summative evaluation. The latter is likely to take place at the end of a period of nursing intervention using a particular nursing model, and involves an exploration of the extent to which the chosen model of nursing proved appropriate to meeting patients' overall needs. As a result of this, it might be found, for example, that certain nursing models are more (or less) appropriate for the care of patients in particular nursing settings.

The Role of the Nurse   A final way in which models of nursing differ from one another is in terms of what they argue should be the role of the nurse in patient care. Whether this should be a 'physician's assistant', a 'patient's advocate', a 'constant presence', a 'facilitator of self-care' or a 'modifier of behavioural patterns' has been a question addressed by many nursing models. However, what remains to be explored more fully is whether certain of these roles might prove to be incompatible with one another, as well as their relative emphasis within different models of nursing. What is certain is that nursing models can not be regarded as neutral in what they have to say about the role of the nurse. The amount of shared decision-making advocated by a model or, alternatively, its emphasis with respect to controlling aspects of nursing is something that can not be ignored.

Nursing Theory

The distinction between models of nursing and nursing theory is not a simple one, since both of these notions have certain features in common. Chinn and Jacobs (1983) define a nursing theory as '. . . A set of concepts, definitions and propositions that projects a systematic view of phenomena by designating specific inter-relationships among concepts for purposes of describing, explaining, predicting and/or controlling phenomena . . .'. Such a definition emphasises that nursing theories, like conceptual models of nursing, are built up out of ideas and concepts. It also emphasises the existence of systematic relationships between these. In these two ways, therefore, theories of nursing would seem to have some

8

affinity with nursing models. However, by claiming that theories attempt to explain and *predict* phenomena, Chinn and Jacobs identify a major source of difference between conceptual models of nursing and nursing theories, the latter being more powerful in what they claim to do.

Moreover, according to Fawcett (1984), while conceptual models are abstract, theories are specific, and their concepts and the relationships between these are more clearly defined. In her earlier writing Fawcett (1978) also claimed that nursing theories should have something to say about what she identifies as four central elements in nursing: the person receiving nursing care; the environment within which the person exists; the nature of the health–illness continuum on which the person falls at the time of interaction with the nurse; and the type of nursing actions deemed appropriate to secure a return to relative well-being.

As may now be apparent, nursing theories are hard to come by. Few nurses would claim that their research has unearthed findings with either the power to explain behaviour comprehensively or the ability to say something about each of the four aspects of patient care which Fawcett identifies as central to nursing. Still less has it been claimed that nurses can predict human behaviour accurately. Instead, nursing today is perhaps best characterised by a variety of theoretical stances, each saying rather different things about people and their care-related needs.

Conceptual models of nursing would seem to exist, therefore, as the starting point for the development of nursing theory. They are not theories themselves, although they may contain the seeds of future ones. It may be useful, therefore, to think of nursing theories as tested and trusted nursing models: powerful ones that have the ability to explain a great deal about what is likely to make effective nursing care.

Having clarified some of the differences between the nursing process, nursing models and nursing theory, it is appropriate to look in detail at a number of conceptual models of nursing. In doing this, the framework identified earlier will be used, and particular attention will be given to models of nursing that make rather different assumptions about people and their nursing needs.

In Chapter 2 this exploration will begin by looking at an approach to care which, while likely to be familiar, does not originate from the insights of nurses or nurse theorists—the *medical model* of care.

After this, two nursing models will be looked at which borrow extensively from the medical model in terms of how they seek to understand people and their health-related needs: the models of nursing suggested by Virginia Henderson and by Nancy Roper, Alison Tierney and Winifred Logan.

Then there will be a consideration of three models of nursing that pay greater attention to psychological and social needs, while not ignoring the existence of physiological mechanisms within people. These will be the nursing models developed by Dorothy Johnson, by Callista Roy and by Dorothea Orem.

Finally, there will be an exploration of two models of nursing that attempt more radical departures from dominant ways of seeing patients and nursing care. Joan Riehl's model of nursing emphasises the human capacity to 'philosophise' and make sense of situations, arguing that nurses should pay particular attention to this in their planning and delivery of care. Martha Rogers's holistic model of nursing works with an unconventional and intellectually challenging view of the relationship between people and their environments, presenting us with a controversial and thought-provoking approach to care.

2

The Medical Model of Care

Introduction

In Chapter 1 it was suggested that some nurses might welcome the introduction of nursing models because these may offer understandings about people which are distinct from those offered by the medical, natural and social sciences.

Before we examine a number of nursing models in detail, therefore, a brief account will be given of the medical model of care—one which will be familiar to most nurses, in that it has for many years formed the basis not only of medical training, but of most nurse training as well.

In an interesting account of the development of medical science Fitzpatrick (1983) has argued that what counts as good medicine and valid medical knowledge varies historically. Before the eighteenth century, medical practice had been largely holistic, with diagnoses and interventions being carefully referenced to the relationship existing between patients and their environments. A recently developed nursing model—that of Martha Rogers (see Chapter 9)—also works with a similar emphasis on holism, considering the overall relationship between people and their environments to be a major factor in influencing health needs.

Current medical science, however, has rejected such approaches and has concentrated on identifying *anatomical*, *physiological* and *biochemical* causes of ill-health. Indeed, the study of anatomy and physiology still dominates much initial medical training today, and among practising doctors the causes of ill-health often come to be identified with imbalances or defects within either, or both, of these

11

aspects of human functioning. However, such modern-day under-standings of the purpose and practice of medicine can have unfortunate consequences. As Kennedy (1983) has recently pointed out, one of these is their tendency to underemphasise political, social and economic forces in the determination of ill-health.

To aid a fuller appreciation of the medical model of care and to facilitate a comparison between it and the nursing models that follow, it may be useful to examine it in more detail, using the framework identified in Chapter 1.

Key Components of Care

The Nature of People

According to the medical model, a person is a complex set of anatomical parts (the lungs, liver, heart, etc.) and physiological systems (the respiratory system, the cardiovascular system, etc.). Within the medical model, much of a person's social behaviour and many of a person's psychological processes are thought to originate from physiological and biochemical activity. While the detailed workings of the mechanisms involved in this activity may be poorly understood at the present time, the medical model argues that many complex psychological and social behaviours can ultimately be explained by biological mechanisms. Such a reductionist view is considered inadequate, not only by many social scientists, but also increasingly by many nurses and some doctors, since it encourages an understanding of people as 'passive hosts of disease' (Reynolds, 1985).

The Causes of Problems Likely to Require Intervention

The medical model emphasises the existence of biological needs within people. As Thibodeau (1983) has suggested, it provides a disease-orientated approach to care which stresses the structure and function of the body rather than the uniqueness of the individual. Thus, both physical and psychological health-care problems are

12

seen as arising when there is a malfunction within either an anatomical part of the body or a physiological system.

Burton (1985) has argued that '. . . Seeing people in these physical terms biases the way health and illness are understood, the way in which the various causes of illness are given different emphases and finally the way in which treatments and preventions are developed . . .'.

The Nature of the Assessment Process

Assessment within the medical model is designed to determine what is *medically* wrong with a person. It therefore focuses on signs and symptoms which are usually elicited by taking a medical history and by physically examining the person in an attempt to identify those physiological systems or anatomical parts which are disturbed in their functioning. Ultimately, the process of assessment will lead to a diagnosis being made. This diagnosis will usually be recognised as a medical 'condition'.

The Nature of the Planning and Goal-setting Process

Once assessment is complete, doctors and nurses working with the medical model plan care to bring about change in particular physiological systems or anatomical parts. Frequently set goals include the restoration of previous levels of balance within particular systems or the return of function within particular parts. In contrast to many of the nursing models that follow, goal-setting is rarely patient-centred. Rather it involves agents (usually doctors) deciding what is the best strategy by which malfunction within a system or part might most effectively be cured.

The Focus of Intervention During the Implementation of the Care Plan

Intervention within the medical model centres on 'putting things right' (Burton, 1985). Thus, it focuses not on the whole person but on the particular physiological system or anatomical part which is perceived to have malfunctioned. As such, it often advocates prescribing and administering medication or removing some anatomical part.

The choice of intervention for a particular patient will depend both on the doctor's past experience of similar 'cases' and on the differences and needs of the individual. However, the medical model tends to stress the importance of the former. Some interventions, or treatments, are so well established that doctors vary little in what they recommend. Others are less so, and considerable variation in treatment may be encountered. It may often be difficult for patients to recognise whether a particular treatment is well established or not.

The Nature of the Process of Evaluating the Quality and Effects of the Care Given

In the medical model, formative evaluation takes place by exploring the extent to which interventions have been successful in meeting goals set for each physiological system or anatomical part deemed to have a malfunction. Summative evaluation of the medical model seems less common, but should involve a consideration of the extent to which the model has been appropriate in meeting a particular set of health-care needs.

The Role of the Nurse

Nurses working with the medical model may find themselves little more than accessories to doctors. Hall (1983) has suggested that efforts by nurses to improve standards of care should be viewed as a positive move towards enhancing nursing's contribution to health-care provision. She further argues that while nurses should in no way 'seek to erode the proper role of medical practitioners', they should not regard themselves as 'physicians' assistants'.

Traditionally, the training of both doctors and nurses has centred around the medical model. However, the usefulness of such a model is increasingly being questioned, not only by nurses, but by some doctors as well. Indeed, Black *et al.* (1984) have suggested that the nature of medicine has been under critical examination for

14

the past twenty years, in terms of both its effectiveness and its role within society.

Faulkner (1985) has suggested that a move away from the medical model of care can be facilitated for nurses by a wider use of the nursing process. However, as has been pointed out, the nursing process alone does not provide nurses with a set of understandings about people and their health-related needs around which to plan and deliver care. This stems from the fact that while the nursing process suggests that nurses should assess, plan, intervene and evaluate, it does not indicate *what* should be the focus of such activities. Nursing models, however, do this when used in conjunction with the nursing process, since they focus the attention on specific aspects of people and their care-related needs. It is this bringing together of nursing models and the nursing process which subsequent chapters seek to explore.

3

Henderson's Model of Nursing

Introduction

In this chapter one of the most well-known models of nursing will be examined—that developed in the work of Virginia Henderson. Like the medical model of care described in Chapter 2, Henderson's model of nursing emphasises the existence of biological needs within people. As will be seen, however, unlike the former, Henderson's nursing model also argues that people have important psychological and social needs that can sometimes lead to a need for nursing care.

In her writing Henderson (1966) acknowledges a number of formative influences on her work. In particular, her belief that nurses need to pay particular attention to accurately interpreting both verbal and non-verbal information from their patients reflects Henderson's appreciation of aspects of behaviourist and interactionist psychology. Furthermore, the work of Wiedenbach (1964), in suggesting the need for a deliberative approach to nursing care, also influenced the development of Henderson's own approach to nursing. As with the medical model of care, her nursing model will be analysed in terms of what it has to say about the seven aspects of people and nursing care identified in Chapter 1.

17

Key Components of Care

The Nature of People

According to Henderson, individuals are best seen as human beings who share certain fundamental human needs: '. . . Whether the person is well or sick the nurse should bear in mind the inescapable human desire for food, shelter, clothing; for love and approval; for a sense of usefulness and mutual dependency in social relationships. . .'. She elaborates further upon this theme, by identifying fourteen fundamental needs common to all individuals (Table 3.1). Under conditions of positive health and well-being, people are likely to have little difficulty in satisfying these needs by themselves. However, in times of illness and at certain points in the life cycle (in childhood, pregnancy and old age, for example), or when death is approaching, an individual may be unable to satisfy these requirements without assistance from others. It is upon such occasions that the unique function of nurses may come into play, as they assist '. . . the individual, sick or well, in the performance of those activities contributing to health or its recovery (or to peaceful death) that he would perform unaided if he had the necessary strength, will or knowledge . . .'.

Table 3.1 Fundamental needs shared by all persons

(1) To breathe normally
(2) To eat and drink adequately
(3) To eliminate body waste
(4) To move and maintain desirable postures
(5) To sleep and rest
(6) To select suitable clothes—dress and undress
(7) To maintain body temperature within normal range
(8) To keep the body clean and well groomed
(9) To avoid changes in the environment; avoid injuring others
(10) To communicate with others
(11) To worship according to one's faith
(12) To work in such a way that there is a sense of accomplishment
(13) To play or participate in forms of recreation
(14) To learn, discover and satisfy curiosity

At all times, nursing care should take place in order to help the person regain independence as rapidly as possible. Henderson calls nursing activities relating to each of these needs components of basic nursing. She identifies fourteen such sets of nursing activities, one relating to each basic need.

The Causes of Problems Likely to Require Nursing Intervention

According to Henderson, nursing care is needed whenever a person is unable to carry out activities contributing to health, recovery or peaceful death. Special difficulties, however, may be associated with particular stages in the life cycle. The very young and the very old, for example, may be unable to satisfy certain of their basic needs because of physical, psychological or social factors associated with their stage of development.

Similarly, temperament and emotional state may also have an effect on a person's ability to satisfy basic human needs. For example, an anxious and fearful patient may experience problems eating, drinking, sleeping and communicating.

Further difficulties may be created by the social and cultural status of the individual. An elderly person, recently bereaved and living alone, may have difficulty in moving around the house, selecting suitable clothing and communicating in the absence of help and support previously provided by a relative or friend.

Finally, physical and intellectual capacities may affect an individual's ability to carry out activities to satisfy basic needs. For example, the mentally and physically handicapped, as well as those who may have lost a special sense or motor capacity, may require nursing care in order to help them to satisfy fundamental needs.

Physical, psychological and social factors such as these limit the individual's ability to carry out activities that lead to the recovery of health. To some extent, they can be seen as creating perceptual, cognitive or behavioural 'sets', dispositions limiting the expression of human potential. Nursing care is, therefore, needed to make 'whole' or 'complete' those needs that are unfilled.

The Nature of the Assessment Process

While Henderson (1972) does not explicitly recommend the use of the nursing process, she argues that the assessment of patient needs

19

should involve negotiation between patient and nurse: '. . . Only in highly dependent states, such as coma or extreme prostration, is the nurse justified in deciding for, rather than with the patient, what is good for him . . .'. She further advocates an empathetic approach to assessment, in which the nurse tries to understand the situation from the patient's point of view. While she does not explicitly argue for it, it would seem that the use of her model with the nursing process would call for a two-stage assessment. In the first part of this, the nurse might work with the patient, considering in turn each fundamental need that might (or might not) be satisfied at present. Between them, they must decide, for each of these needs, whether nursing assistance is needed. After this, they may move to a second stage of assessment in which decisions are made as to the causes of problems relating to specific demands for nursing care. These may be related to age, temperament, social and cultural status, or present physical or intellectual capacity.

The Nature of the Planning and Goal-setting Process

Henderson advocates that in many nursing situations long-term goals will relate to helping the patient to regain independence with respect to fundamental human needs. Short-term and intermediate goals may also be set along the way. These should relate to the causes of problems identified during assessment, and are also likely to take into account the presence of pathological states or syndromes such as shock, fever, infection or dehydration. A written care plan, modified in the light of the outcome of nursing interventions identified within it, is recommended.

The Focus of Intervention During the Implementation of the Care Plan

With Henderson's model, nursing intervention takes the form of nursing actions aimed at achieving long-term intermediate and short-term goals. A series of these are likely to be specified within the plan of nursing care, relating to each area of human need in which a deficiency has been identified.

Since Henderson believes that nursing care is something to be carried out in close conjunction with that provided by medically qualified personnel, the plan of nursing care should explicitly include drugs and treatments prescribed by the physician. In this respect, Henderson's model of nursing differs from some others to be described, in that it explicitly acknowledges this complementary relationship between nursing and medical care.

Finally, it is important to recognise that successful nursing interventions may also require the involvement of the patient's family and other members of the health-care team.

The Nature of the Process of Evaluating the Quality and Effects of the Care Given

With this model of nursing, the final stage of the nursing process— evaluation—is likely to take place through an examination of the extent to which the patient has been helped by the nurse to meet basic needs that were in some way unmet before nursing intervention took place.

Ideally, evaluation should involve an enquiry into the extent to which goals, agreed upon between patient and nurse, have been met. Such formative evaluation provides the means by which the nurse may revise the plan of care drawn up for a particular patient. Summative evaluation may be carried out over a number of weeks and with a number of patients, aiming to evaluate the overall usefulness of Henderson's model of nursing within a particular nursing setting.

The Role of the Nurse

Henderson (1966) describes two rather different roles for the nurse which fit rather uneasily together. On the one hand, she stresses the unique function of the nurse as an independent health-care professional. In this role, she advocates a complementary role for nursing in seeking to substitute 'for what the patient lacks to make him complete, whole, [and] independent'. However, she also identifies a more stereotyped nursing role, that of physician's helper, with the allied possibility of nursing goals being subsumed within a medical plan of treatment.

21

More recently, Fitzpatrick and Whall (1983) have suggested that Henderson, like Florence Nightingale, views nature as the ultimate curer of disease. This being so, they argue that Henderson sees the role of the nurse as that of an intermediary between person and environment.

Using Henderson's Model with the Nursing Process

As has been suggested, the Henderson model of nursing is perhaps one of the most familiar to practising nurses today. Nevertheless, some suggestions will be made about its use with the nursing process in planning and delivering care. It should be borne in mind, however, that, since Henderson's model of nursing works with a firm commitment to patient participation in care, this is likely to have implications for all stages of the nursing process.

Assessment—First Stage

The first stage of the process of patient assessment is likely to identify those fundamental needs that are not being met. In most instances nurse and patient should reach agreement about these, the nurse only deciding on behalf of patients when they are unable to participate in the process.

For example, a nurse working in a hospital may observe that a particular child is unwilling to eat or drink. If information subsequently gained from the parents indicates that this is unusual behaviour for the person concerned, then, as the first stage in the assessment, the nurse may decide that for this individual the need to eat or drink is not being satisfied.

Alternatively, following a rib injury, a patient may complain of increased awareness of the need to breathe. In such a case the nurse and patient may assess the need to breathe normally as being only partly met.

Assessment—Second Stage

Once the areas of chief concern have been identified and the relevant fundamental needs highlighted, the nurse will proceed to

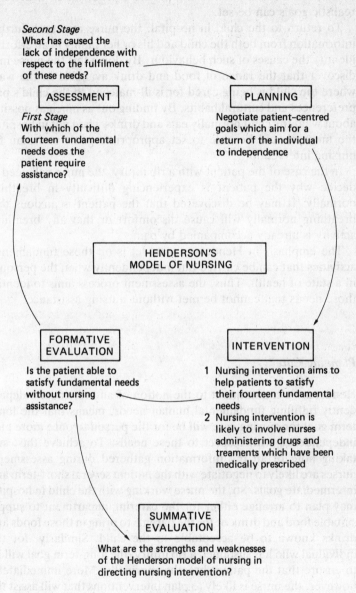

Second Stage
What has caused the
lack of independence with
respect to the fulfilment
of these needs?

ASSESSMENT

PLANNING

First Stage
With which of the
fourteen fundamental
needs does the
patient require
assistance?

Negotiate patient-centred
goals which aim for a
return of the individual
to independence

HENDERSON'S
MODEL OF NURSING

FORMATIVE
EVALUATION

INTERVENTION

Is the patient able to
satisfy fundamental needs
without nursing
assistance?

1 Nursing intervention aims to
help patients to satisfy
their fourteen fundamental
needs
2 Nursing intervention is
likely to involve nurses
administering drugs and
treaments which have been
medically prescribed

SUMMATIVE
EVALUATION

What are the strengths and weaknesses
of the Henderson model of nursing in
directing nursing intervention?

Figure 3.1

the second stage of the assessment process. Here the aim will be to decide the likely causes of the patient's problems in order that realistic goals can be set.

To return to the child in hospital: the nurse may seek further information from both the child and his or her family in an effort to identify the causes of such behaviour. By doing this the nurse may discover that the range of food and drink available in the ward where the child is being cared for is ill-matched to the child's past preferences and cultural habits. By finding out as much as possible about what the child normally eats and drinks when not in hospital, the nurse should be able to set appropriate goals and plan for nursing intervention.

In the case of the patient with a rib injury, the nurse will need to decide why the patient is experiencing difficulty in breathing normally. It may be discovered that the patient is anxious that breathing normally will cause discomfort or that any breathing activity is already accompanied by pain.

The emphasis in Henderson's model is on those fundamental activities that can be carried out independently when the person is in a state of health. Thus, the assessment process aims to identify those needs that cannot be met without nursing assistance.

Planning Care

Henderson's commitment to the notion of an individual independently fulfilling fundamental human needs, means that the long-term goal for nursing care will be for the person to once more gain independence with respect to these needs. To achieve this, and taking note of all the information gathered during assessment, nurses are likely to negotiate with the patient several short-term and intermediate goals. So, the nurse working with the child in hospital may plan to arrange either for the catering department to supply suitable food and drink or for the parents to bring in those foods and drinks known to be acceptable to the child. Similarly, for the individual who has sustained a rib injury, the long-term goal will be to ensure that the patient breathes normally. More immediately, however, the nurse is likely to plan interventions that will assist the patient to breathe more easily. This may involve setting goals related to relieving the patient's anxiety or relieving the patient's present level of pain.

Patient-centred goals set while planning care should be realistic and should look forward to the evaluation stage of the nursing process by identifying those behaviours that may later be observed and measured to evaluate the success (or otherwise) of nursing intervention.

Nursing Intervention and the Delivery of Care

Henderson's model of nursing is not very explicit with respect to recommended nursing interventions, although Adam (1980) has suggested a number of ways of intervening that may be appropriate for use with this model. These include positively reinforcing the patient, completing tasks for him and increasing the supply of factors needed for recovery to health. Certainly, while Henderson accepts the idea that nursing should take place side by side with medical intervention, the activities that nurses might engage in are not readily identified. What follows, therefore, is an attempt to suggest appropriate interventions that seem to meet the demand within the model for goals that aim to help the patient to achieve independence.

Henderson's model takes into account the constraints imposed by age on achieving independence. Thus, it would be unrealistic for nursing interventions to seek to achieve complete independence for a young child. While acknowledging that family members have a role to play in the delivery of care, Henderson remains relatively non-explicit about the manner in which they might contribute to this. Nursing intervention, therefore, will take place to ensure that adequate food and drink is available for the child, but no greater degree of independence on the part of the child will be sought for.

In the case of the patient with a rib injury, the nurse may intervene to verbally encourage him to appreciate that breathing might not be as painful as he imagines. An attempt may also be made to remain with the patient until some reduction in his overall level of anxiety has been achieved. Alternatively, if the patient is experiencing pain, the nurse may suggest a more comfortable position in which to rest or may administer forms of medication prescribed by the physician.

Evaluation

In formatively evaluating the care given to patients, nurses are likely to use their care plans to determine how far the goals set at the planning stage have been met. Nurses working with Henderson's model of nursing, in particular, are likely to begin a formative evaluation of their care by re-examining each fundamental need diagnosed during assessment as being incompletely met by the person's own resources. The nurse will then look at the extent to which goals relating to each need have been satisfied. For every unsatisfied goal, new nursing interventions may be identified, or the goal itself may be reformulated to allow a greater potential for success in subsequent nursing care.

Thus, the nurse caring for the young child is likely to search for evidence of a return to a more normal pattern of eating and drinking for that child. In order to achieve a more precise evaluation, the nurse may record the child's dietary intake over a number of days.

Evidence of goal attainment for the person with a rib injury may be gained by questioning the patient about the ease with which breathing takes place following nursing intervention. It may also involve the observation of those activities that the patient is subsequently able to achieve without becoming breathless or uncomfortable.

Summative evaluation of Henderson's model of nursing can only take place after it has been worked with for some time in a particular nursing context. In carrying out this type of evaluation, nurses are likely to explore the effectiveness of this particular model of care, compared with others, in meeting the needs of a wide range of patients in that particular setting. Nurses may also want to enquire whether working with this particular nursing model gives them sufficient autonomy as members of the health-care team, or whether the conception of nurse role which it advocates renders them insufficiently independent in the management of patient care.

4

Roper, Logan and Tierney's Activities of Living Model of Nursing

Introduction

One of the most familiar models of nursing to practising nurses in Britain is that originally devised by Roper (1976) and subsequently elaborated upon in work by Roper, Logan and Tierney (1980, 1981, 1983). Like Henderson's model of nursing, the one proposed by these writers has been widely used in a variety of nursing settings.

Roper's early work laid the foundations for this model of nursing by attempting to bring together a variety of insights from the study of physiology, psychology and nursing. In doing this, she sought first of all to identify a number of key qualities common to all human beings. In carrying out such a task, Roper believed that it was essential to focus on the observable behaviours that accompany these qualities, since she believed that a rigorous approach to nursing should be based upon observable and measurable phenomena and not upon intuition or good luck in the planning and delivery of care.

As with other models, Roper, Logan and Tierney's model of nursing will be examined in terms of what it has to say about seven key aspects of people and nursing. Then an attempt will be made to explore how this model might be used in conjunction with the nursing process.

Key Components of Care

The Nature of People

According to Roper, Logan and Tierney's model of nursing, one of the best ways to understand people is in terms of the activities they perform. Roper herself originally identified sixteen *Activities of Daily Living* (ADL). Some of these are behaviours essential for the maintenance of life. Others increase the quality of life but are not essential for it. One (dying) is singled out for special attention, since it is the final act of living a person engages in. These sixteen Activities of Daily Living are shown in Table 4.1.

This catalogue of behaviours has subsequently been revised by Roper and her colleagues to specify twelve *Activities of Living* (AL), each of which refers to a relatively distinct type of human behaviour. These twelve activities are further said to be related to

Table 4.1   Activities of Daily Living

Essential	Breathing
	Eating
	Eliminating
	Controlling body temperature
	Mobilising
	Sleeping
	Fulfilling safety and security needs
Increase quality of living	Personal cleansing
	Dressing
	Communicating
	Learning
	Working
	Playing
	Sexualising
	Procreating
Mortality	Dying

28

particular human needs. Indeed, they are simply the behavioural manifestations of these. Table 4.2 lists the twelve Activities of Living identified in more recent versions of this nursing model.

Some of these Activities of Living have a biological basis to them. Others, such as those relating to personal dress, cleanliness, the nature of work and play, and sexuality, have social and cultural determinants. In addition, Roper, Logan and Tierney argue that individuals differ from one another in the ways in which they involve themselves in Activities of Living. To some extent, such variations can be related to the age of the person concerned, with both young and elderly people being less independent in their performance of a variety of Activities of Living. Differences between individuals in the expression of Activities of Living can also result from differences in past social and cultural experience. Some people may not involve themselves in the expression of certain Activities of Living through personal choice; others, through lack of social or cultural opportunity.

Table 4.2   Activities of Living

---

(1) Maintaining a safe environment
(2) Communicating
(3) Breathing
(4) Eating and drinking
(5) Eliminating
(6) Personal cleansing and dressing
(7) Controlling body temperature
(8) Mobilising
(9) Working and playing
(10) Expressing sexuality
(11) Sleeping
(12) Dying

More tentatively, Roper, Logan and Tierney have identified a further three types of activity that humans can involve themselves in. They call these *preventing*, *comforting* and *seeking* behaviours. These terms describe broad patterns of behaviour available to both nurses and patients throughout the caring process.

The Causes of Problems Likely to Require Nursing Intervention

Roper, Logan and Tierney's model of nursing identifies a number of different situations which may call for nursing care. The model suggests that childhood, pregnancy and old age may call for nursing intervention related to particular activities at these stages of life which can only be accomplished with help from other people. Other more transitory conditions may also call for nursing care. Roper, Logan and Tierney identify five main sets of factors that can give rise to such needs: disability and disturbed physiology; pathological and degenerative tissue change; accident; infection; and effects arising from a person's physical, psychological or social environment.

Such conditions may move the individual from a state of relative independence to one of relative dependence for a particular Activity of Living.

The Nature of the Assessment Process

Roper, Logan and Tierney's model of nursing suggests that Activities of Living can be used as a basis around which an assessment of individual needs can be carried out. Assessment is likely to involve the nurse and patient in considering each activity in turn, identifying previous routines, coping mechanisms and actual, or potential, nursing problems. Sometimes it may involve a consideration of all the Activities of Living specified by the model. On other occasions the nurse may use insight into available nursing actions to focus in the short term more specifically upon certain Activities of Living. It should be noted, however, that this model of nursing strongly advocates continuing assessment with respect to patient needs.

The Nature of the Planning and Goal-setting process

Once a series of goals have been negotiated between patient and nurse, the latter's attention should be turned to the resources that are available for nursing care. A consideration of the environment and the availability of personnel and equipment is likely to suggest a number of alternative strategies that could be used in patient care.

30

Roper, Logan and Tierney argue, however, that the process of selecting between alternative strategies should be carried out on an informed basis and not simply in accordance with past precedent in that particular nursing context.

The Focus of Intervention During the Implementation of the Care Plan

Implementation of the care plan can take place once the nurse has selected the most appropriate nursing actions from those available. In trying to achieve the goals that have been previously negotiated with the patient, nurses may use a variety of actions related to the particular Activities of Living with which the patient is experiencing difficulty. Thus, intervention may be made in order to ensure adequate mobility or restfulness, or to allow effective communication and learning to take place. Many nursing actions are likely to involve the three broad patterns of response identified earlier. Thus, nurses may act to *prevent* certain situations arising. They may *comfort* the patient both physically and mentally. Alternatively, they may try to minimise the dependence of the patient so as to allow of a fuller expression of desires to *seek* responsibility for self-care.

The Nature of the Process of Evaluating the Quality and Effects of the Care Given

According to Roper, Logan and Tierney, patient behaviours decided upon at the planning and goal-setting stage of the nursing process should be the criteria used in formative evaluation. Evaluation of care, therefore, is likely to require a comparison, for each Activity of Living, between observable behaviour before and after nursing intervention. When expected outcomes do not take place, the patient and nurse should reassess that particular area of difficulty.

Summative evaluation, on the other hand, should also take place to explore the value of the Roper, Logan and Tierney model in particular care settings. Evaluation of this type is likely to take place once a number of nurses have worked with the model and, hence, when the results of several formative evaluations are available.

31

When nursing situations are encountered in which the Roper, Logan and Tierney model proves to be of limited value, an overall summative evaluation may suggest the use of alternative models of nursing.

The Role of the Nurse

Roper, Logan and Tierney (1980) have described the caring and comforting role of the nurse as one which sees the nurse acting as an *independent* practitioner. They further argue that this is the role most often taken on by nurses today. However, they also suggest that nurses may take on a more *dependent* role, assisting doctors with procedures that aim to either alleviate or cure medical conditions. Additionally, they identify a further *interdependent* role—that adopted by nurses when they work with other members of the health-care team.

Using Roper, Logan and Tierney's Model of Nursing with the Nursing Process

Some of the main features of the model of nursing developed by Roper, Logan and Tierney having been described, suggestions will now be made about how it might be put into practice with the nursing process.

Assessment

Roper, Logan and Tierney express a firm commitment to the idea of a continuous process of assessment in nursing care. By repeatedly reassessing patients and their needs, nurses are likely to be able to gain greater insight into the nature of problems affecting those in their care. Thus, it would seem appropriate to consider assessment as a continuing part of the nursing process rather than as an activity that can be divided into discrete stages.

According to the Roper, Logan and Tierney model, nursing assessment should focus on the individual's ability to carry out the

32

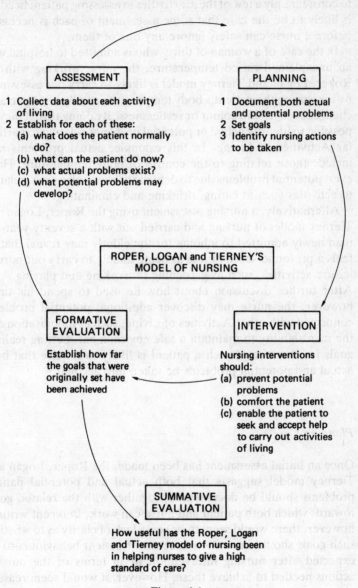

ASSESSMENT

1 Collect data about each activity of living
2 Establish for each of these:
   (a) what does the patient normally do?
   (b) what can the patient do now?
   (c) what actual problems exist?
   (d) what potential problems may develop?

PLANNING

1 Document both actual and potential problems
2 Set goals
3 Identify nursing actions to be taken

ROPER, LOGAN and TIERNEY'S MODEL OF NURSING

FORMATIVE EVALUATION

Establish how far the goals that were originally set have been achieved

INTERVENTION

Nursing interventions should:
   (a) prevent potential problems
   (b) comfort the patient
   (c) enable the patient to seek and accept help to carry out activities of living

SUMMATIVE EVALUATION

How useful has the Roper, Logan and Tierney model of nursing been in helping nurses to give a high standard of care?

Figure 4.1

33

twelve Activities of Living. While Roper, Logan and Tierney have suggested that there are circumstances when it might be appropriate to consider only a few of these activities in assessing patient needs, it is likely to be the case that some assessment of each is necessary before a nurse can safely ignore any one of them.

In the case of a woman of thirty who is admitted to hospital with an unexplained raised temperature, the nurse working with the Roper, Logan and Tierney model is likely to carry out assessment by measuring the patient's body temperature and by noting related changes such as skin colour or restlessness. By doing this, it may be possible to identify actual or potential problems relating to particular Activities of Living. In this example, actual problems may include those relating to the control of body temperature. However, potential problems due to dehydration may also exist, relating to activities such as eating, drinking and eliminating.

Alternatively, a nursing assessment using the Roper, Logan and Tierney model of nursing and carried out with a seventy-year-old man newly admitted to a home for the elderly may reveal that he feels a profound sense of loss at being unable to carry out normal leisure activities, such as gardening (a working and playing AL). After further discussion about how he used to spend his time, however, the nurse may discover additional potential problems connected with other Activities of Living, such as mobilisation and the man's ability to maintain a safe environment. Setting realistic goals for the care of such a patient is likely to require that both actual and potential problems be taken into account.

Planning Care

Once an initial assessment has been made, the Roper, Logan and Tierney model suggests that both actual and potential patient problems should be documented, together with the related goals towards which both patient and nurse can work. In recent writing, however, there would seem to be some lack of clarity as to whether such goals should be written in terms of patient behaviours to be expected after nursing intervention or in terms of the nursing actions needed to achieve these. However, it would seem reasonable to recommend the adoption of the former course of action, as this preserves the notion of patient-centred care and aids a subsequent evaluation of this.

Thus, in the first example cited, the long-term goal might be that the woman's ability to control her temperature will be restored. In the short-term, however, nursing interventions may be planned to avoid potential problems associated with Activities of Living such as eating, drinking and eliminating. In the case of the elderly man, the nurse may negotiate with him what leisure activities would be acceptable within the home for the elderly to which he has been admitted. By careful planning it may be possible to link the attainment of these goals to those related to mobility and the maintenance of a safe environment.

By encouraging nurses to consider available resources and personnel in planning care, the Roper, Logan and Tierney model emphasises the role that other health-care professionals can play in patient-care. Thus, the advice and help of both a physiotherapist and an occupational therapist may be sought in an effort to set realistic goals for the elderly man.

Nursing Intervention and the Delivery of Care

Once patient-centred goals have been agreed, the implementation of the care plan can begin. The Roper, Logan and Tierney model argues that nursing interventions should focus on the patient's normal routines, thereby minimising any anxiety that might be caused by a drastic change in habits. As has already been mentioned, nursing intervention can take place in one of three ways: preventing, comforting and responding to patients who seek nursing help. It may also include activities such as those associated with the administration of medications, and the carrying out of dressings and investigations.

In the case of the woman with a raised temperature, nursing intervention may take the form of explanation and comfort during the period of medical investigation associated with this. In addition, the nurse may aim to prevent the development of potential problems identified during assessment. Similarly, the elderly man may require comforting to help him cope with the loss of his normal routine. Nurses and others involved in his care may seek to involve

35

him in a different range of activities from those to which he had previously been accustomed; introducing him to new leisure pursuits, while retaining as much of his former life-style as possible. By introducing activities in which the man is able to participate, the nurse may be successful in preventing both boredom and physical and mental deterioration.

Keeping a record of the nursing interventions carried out is an essential feature of Roper, Logan and Tierney's model of nursing and is recommended both for the benefit of the patient and to facilitate the development of nursing knowledge.

Evaluation

The starting point for evaluation should be the goals originally set during the planning of nursing care. Following a specified period of nursing intervention, each Activity of Living should be re-examined to establish whether or not the goal set has been achieved. In carrying out such formative evaluation, nurses are likely to use similar skills to those employed during assessment: measurement, observation and discussion.

Thus, in evaluating the care of the woman of thirty with the raised temperature, the nurse is likely to explore not only whether her temperature has returned to normal, but also whether the potential problem of dehydration has been avoided. To do this, it may be necessary to measure her urinary output, observe her skin condition and talk with her to ascertain whether or not she feels thirsty.

Similarly, the nurse may be able to evaluate the quality of the elderly man's nursing care by observing the Activities of Living that he is able to involve himself in after nursing intervention. By so doing, the nurse may discover whether the comfort supplied has helped him adapt to a different life-style.

Summative evaluation of the Roper, Logan and Tierney model of nursing should involve an exploration of the extent to which it seems able to provide sensitive and appropriate standards of nursing within a given speciality or area of care. In particular, nurses may wish to explore the extent to which this particular model assigns nurses a role in patient-care different from that provided by doctors and other health-care personnel.

5

Johnson's Behavioural Systems Model of Nursing

Introduction

Both Henderson's and Roper, Logan and Tierney's models of nursing emphasise the interaction between biological, psychological and social factors as influences on human behaviour. They differ from each other, however, in terms of the relative emphasis they give to each of these influences as factors to be taken into account in planning and delivering nursing care. Furthermore, it can be argued that by failing to analyse in detail the ways in which such factors interact to affect behaviour in ill-health, both of these models encourage a tacit acceptance of the types of explanation offered by the medical model of care.

In contrast to such nursing models, that proposed by Johnson (1980) attempts a radical move away from medical understandings of people and their needs in health and illness. The Johnson Behavioural Systems model of nursing was developed at the University of California in the late 1960s and early 1970s, and is a model of nursing which encourages those working with it to focus on the types of *behaviour* that people can display, rather than on needs that they may have. The details of this nursing model will be explored in terms of what it has to say about seven key aspects of people and nursing care.

Key Components of Care

The Nature of People

The Johnson Behavioural Systems model of nursing encourages nurses to see individuals as having a set of interrelated behavioural sub-systems, each striving for balance and equilibrium within itself. According to the model, there are seven major sub-systems in each person—the affiliative, the achievement, the aggressive, the dependency, the eliminative, the ingestive and the sexual sub-systems. Grubbs (1980) has identified a possible eighth sub-system—the restorative. Each of these sub-systems motivates an individual's behaviour towards particular goals. The relationship between each sub-system and the goal to which it motivates behaviour is shown in Table 5.1.

Furthermore, what Johnson calls the *action* of each sub-system, in striving to attain goals relevant to it, is likely to be limited in a number of ways by the individual's past experience. It may, for

Table 5.1 Johnson's seven behavioural sub-systems and the goals towards which they motivate behaviour

Sub-system	Behaviour motivated
Achievement	Towards control over oneself and one's environment
Affiliative	Towards relationships of intimacy with others
Aggressive	Towards self-protection from threat and towards self-assertion
Dependency	Towards conditions of security and dependency upon others
Eliminative	Towards the expulsion of biological wastes
Ingestive	Towards maintaining the integrity of the organism and towards achieving states of bodily pleasure
Sexual	Towards sexual gratification and towards caring for others

example, be affected by people's perceptions of the behavioural options open to them, by their understandings of what they can and can not do, and by whether or not these perceptions accord with what is truly the case. Johnson suggests that such limitations relate to what she calls a person's *choice* of behaviour. Further constraints on an individual's actions are likely to be imposed by past predispositions towards certain kinds of behaviour. These are what Johnson calls *sets*. She distinguishes between two major types of set: the *preparatory set*, created by actions and objects immediately around the person, and the *perseverative set*, created by past habits.

It is possible to see in this description a number of themes derived from work in the biological and social sciences. The image of the person as a set of balanced sub-systems should be familiar to anyone acquainted with the biological concept of homoeostasis. Furthermore, the tendency for sub-systems within an individual to motivate behaviour towards some sort of goal shares some affinity with the work of both drive theorists such as Hull (1951) and humanistic psychologists such as Maslow (1970) and Rogers (1951). The latter, in particular, claim to have identified tendencies within people which motivate them to strive towards conditions of physiological and psychological equilibrium which allow for personal development and growth.

Moreover, the idea that human motivations can be interfaced with and deflected from their course by processes connected with past learning, fits well with much of the work of social learning theorists such as Bandura (1969). We can, therefore, see in Johnson's image of the person a somewhat eclectic use of insights derived from recent work in the biological and social sciences.

The Causes of Problems Likely to Require Nursing Intervention

According to Johnson's model of nursing, a person's behavioural sub-systems can be thrown into disequilibrium either by processes associated with physical disease or by changes in personal requirements and patterns of daily living. In either case, it is the nurse's task to help disturbed sub-systems back into a condition of balance. This can only be done after first carrying out a nursing assessment of the individual concerned.

The Nature of the Assessment Process

According to Johnson, nursing assessment should be neither haphazard nor intuitive. Instead it needs to be organised around a careful examination of each behavioural sub-system in turn, with the nurse aiming to identify the conditions of relative balance or imbalance within each. According to Grubbs (1980), such a process of assessment is likely to take place in two stages. The first of these enables the nurse to detect those sub-systems that are out of equilibrium. The second stage aims to identify possible causes of such imbalance.

The Nature of the Planning and Goal-setting Process

Next, the nurse working with this model should draw up a care plan based upon the sub-systems examined. Much of the nurse's effort at this stage is likely to be organised around an attempt to provide what Johnson calls the *sustenal imperatives* (what could be regarded as the personal requirements) essential for the growth and return to balance of each sub-system. *Protection*, *nurturance* and *stimulation* are the primary means by which the nurse aims to restore each sub-system to equilibrium, and, in aiming to bring about such changes, *environmental variables* will be manipulated in the process of nursing intervention.

The Focus of Nursing Intervention During the Implementation of the Care Plan

According to Johnson, the nurse may intervene in one of four ways. First, the person may be *restricted* by limits or external controls imposed on behaviour. Second, the individual may be *defended* by the nurse offering protection against external stressors and threats. Third, an attempt may be made to *inhibit* the person by suppressing ineffective responses. Finally, the nurse may *facilitate* the person by offering nurturance and stimulation. Such modes of intervention are likely to be familiar, although the terminology which Johnson uses to describe them may be less so.

The Nature of the Process of Evaluating the Quality and Effects of the Care Given

Evaluation requires the prior setting of long-term, intermediate and short-term goals for each person receiving nursing care. These need to be expressed in terms of behaviours that will be both observable and measurable once they have been achieved. Once this has been done, it will be possible to evaluate the extent to which these kinds of goals have been attained at the end of designated periods of time. As before, it is necessary to distinguish between the on-going or formative evaluation of Johnson's model of nursing and summative evaluation. While the everyday work of all nurses working with the model should involve the former, there will be times when a consideration of the overall appropriateness of Johnson's model as a set of guidelines for care within a particular nursing speciality will also be appropriate.

The Role of the Nurse

Finally, Johnson's model of nursing defines a role for the nurse which is complementary to that of the doctor but not dependent upon it. The model's emphasis upon observable behaviour shows a concern for people rather than their biological functioning. Thus, nursing's distinctive contribution to patient care is through control mechanisms which aim to facilitate optimal levels of behaviour. The role of the nurse therefore becomes one of restoring balance within behavioural sub-systems at times of psychological or physical crisis. It is important to recognise, however, that Johnson has also identified a preventative role for nurses by arguing that health-related problems can be anticipated and avoided.

Using Johnson's Behavioural Systems Model of Nursing with the Nursing Process

While it is beyond the scope of this chapter to examine in detail even one study of nursing care using the Johnson model of nursing, a number of suggestions will be made about how nurses might begin to work with the model in conjunction with the nursing process.

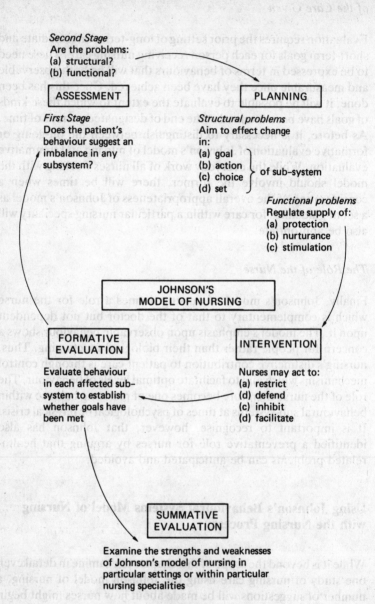

Second Stage
Are the problems:
(a) structural?
(b) functional?

ASSESSMENT

PLANNING

First Stage
Does the patient's
behaviour suggest an
imbalance in any
subsystem?

Structural problems
Aim to effect change
in:
(a) goal
(b) action
(c) choice
(d) set

} of sub-system

Functional problems
Regulate supply of:
(a) protection
(b) nurturance
(c) stimulation

JOHNSON'S
MODEL OF NURSING

FORMATIVE
EVALUATION

INTERVENTION

Evaluate behaviour
in each affected sub-
system to establish
whether goals have
been met

Nurses may act to:
(a) restrict
(d) defend
(c) inhibit
(d) facilitate

SUMMATIVE
EVALUATION

Examine the strengths and weaknesses
of Johnson's model of nursing in
particular settings or within particular
nursing specialities

Figure 5.1

42

Assessment—First Stage

Initially, the nurse aims to discover whether or not a nursing problem exists or might be expected to exist. To achieve this, each sub-system is considered in turn, and, on the basis of the patient's behaviour, the nurse identifies any sub-systems that are in, or likely to be in, disequilibrium.

In the case of a young man attending a psychiatric day clinic and avoiding social contact with both staff and patients, a first-stage assessment might suggest an imbalance within the affiliative sub-system and possibly also in the aggressive sub-system. In other words, the goals of these two sub-systems may not be being met (see Table 5.1).

Another example could be that of an elderly woman suffering from persistent vomiting. Here a first-stage assessment might suggest the presence of disequilibrium in both eliminative and ingestive sub-systems.

Assessment—Second Stage

During the second stage of assessment, a more detailed examination of those sub-systems identified earlier as out of equilibrium is likely to be carried out.

In doing this, Johnson suggests a differentiation should be made between problems that are *structural* within the sub-system and those that are *functional*: that is, arising from the external environment. Thus, during this part of the assessment process, the nurse is likely to seek information to help to decide whether intervention will need to be directed towards alleviating either structural or functional imbalance, or both. To do this, observations are likely to be made of the patient's verbal and non-verbal behaviour, and these will be used to check with the patient the problems identified. Nurses will need to be particularly receptive to information suggesting which sustenal imperatives should be manipulated in order to restore equilibrium.

To return to the two examples: during the second stage of assessment, the nurse would try to determine whether the young man appeared uncommunicative in other, different, settings. This would tend to indicate the existence of a structural problem. If this is the case, plans might be made to extend his range of choice about how to behave with people in small groups. However, by asking relatives and others about his behaviour away from the day centre, the nurse may decide that his apparent withdrawal was specific to that particular context and conclude that the problem was of a functional nature.

In the case of the elderly woman with persistent vomiting, a second-stage assessment might well demonstrate the existence of a functional problem in the eliminative sub-system. This might suggest the need for nursing intervention in the ingestive sub-system, to restrict or limit food intake and to facilitate adequate nourishment by other means. This latter example highlights Johnson's belief that disequilibrium in one sub-system may affect other, interrelated, sub-systems.

Planning Care

Having identified the particular sub-systems that are in disequilibrium, the nurse plans a series of interventions. Long-term goals are likely to be concerned with the maintenance or restoration of balance within and between each sub-system.

If a problem is considered to be structural, the nurse is likely to plan her care to effect change in the goal, set, choice or action of the sub-system. If the problem is functional in nature, then, having determined during assessment the sustenal imperatives that may be insufficient or excessive, the nurse is likely to plan to alter the patient's environment so as to make the supply of these more appropriate.

Following assessment, the nurse may plan a programme of intervention to help to develop the communication skills of the young man in the previous examples, or a decision may be made to introduce him to a different environment—perhaps one with fewer people or with people closer to his own age. Only after a detailed assessment will the nurse know which environmental variables to manipulate.

As was suggested in considering the process of assessment, care planning for the elderly woman might focus upon the ingestive sub-system, even though disequilibrium exists primarily in the eliminative sub-system. An initial plan might involve restriction within the ingestive sub-system with the aim of maintaining hydration via an intravenous infusion, thus facilitating sufficient nourishment while preventing further disequilibrium. In a detailed care plan, a series of short-term and intermediate goals would probably be set, with the overall long-term goal being that of sub-system equilibrium.

Nursing Intervention and the Delivery of Care

According to Johnson, the major aim of nursing intervention is to ensure the fulfilment of the goals of each behavioural sub-system. Thus, having identified problems as either structural or functional in nature, the nurse intervenes to help the patient to achieve short-term, intermediate and long-term goals.

The nurse may intervene in one of four ways. First, patients may be restricted by the nurse suggesting various limitations on behaviour. Thus, the elderly woman with persistent vomiting might only be allowed fluids, or might be restricted to sips of water while receiving fluids parenterally. Second, the nurse may defend the patient from external threats. Thus, the young man might be protected from the stress of coping in a large group. Third, the nurse may inhibit a patient's behaviour by suppressing ineffective responses. Such inhibition would seem more likely to be effective if accompanied by the simultaneous facilitation of other behaviour. Hence, the young man receiving nursing care may make less use of his ineffective behaviour once his choice of responses is extended. The fourth mode of intervention, that of facilitating, might be considered a partner of the third mode in some circumstances. To return to the example of the young man learning communication skills, his ineffective responses may be more inhibited if he is facilitated by stimulation and encouragement to exhibit new behavioural skills.

Evaluation

Johnson suggests that, in order to evaluate nursing care, it is necessary to predict the outcomes that are likely to arise from successful nursing intervention. Moreover, nurses working with this model of nursing should express these outcomes in terms of

45

behaviours that can be observed. Ideally, these should be identified early on in the nursing process, at the stage of setting goals and planning care. Thus, the nurse should consider what behaviours will indicate that nursing intervention has been successful.

It is further argued that this evaluation can take one of two forms. First, there may be expected outcomes within a sub-system. Certain patient behaviours may indicate the success, or otherwise, of nursing interventions in response to structural problems. Second, expected outcomes may be related to environmental variables. Here behavioural changes may have resulted from nursing interventions related to a functional problem.

In evaluating nursing interventions made for the young man receiving psychiatric nursing care, the nurse might expect to see him using some of his newly learned communication skills in situations that he had previously found stressful. He might also be expected to be less withdrawn in small group settings. Similarly, in evaluating the care delivered to the elderly woman with persistent vomiting, the nurse might expect her to vomit less frequently and to show behavioural signs of adequate hydration, such as passing normal amounts of urine.

Evaluation is, however, closely related to reassessment, and, if expected outcomes do not take place, the nurse must reassess the patient within each sub-system. Formative evaluation such as that described is likely to take place as the time set for the attainment of each goal is reached. The nurse, therefore, is likely to assess the patient and evaluate the care given continuously as the care plan is implemented.

Summative evaluation of this nursing model is crucial if nurses are to become more informed about the circumstances in which its use is most appropriate. In carrying out this type of evaluation, nurses should review the total care of those patients who have been nursed according to Johnson's model. In doing this, the aim will be to identify strengths and weaknesses associated with the use of a model of nursing that operates with a notion of interrelated behavioural sub-systems. Over time, it may thereby become possible to evaluate the effectiveness of this particular model in a number of different areas of nursing practice. It may further be possible to identify nursing specialities in which the use of the model seems particularly appropriate.

46

6

Roy's Adaptation Model of Nursing

Introduction

In looking at previous models of nursing, it has been emphasised that, in developing these, nurse theorists have frequently used existing theoretical insights from the biological and social sciences. Because of this, models of nursing often relate to more generally held perspectives about the causes of human behaviour. Such a characteristic is particularly true of the model of nursing devised by Roy (1980, 1984), which seeks to extend Helson's (1964) concept of psychological adaptation to the field of nursing care.

In this chapter the main features of the Roy Adaptation model of nursing will be identified, and a number of suggestions will then be made about how it may be put into practice in the nursing process.

Key Components of Care

The Nature of People

Roy, in a similar way to Johnson (1980), sees people as individuals possessing sets of interrelated systems within them. Her model differs from that of Johnson, however, in that she does not conceptualise these systems in purely behavioural terms. Instead

47

Roy argues that people are best understood as sets of interconnected biological, psychological and social systems that influence behaviour. Because of this emphasis, Roy describes her nursing model as a *bio-psycho-social* model of nursing.

In addition to identifying such systems within the individual, Roy's model of nursing argues that each system exists in a state of constant interaction with the environment, striving to maintain relative balance, both within itself and in its relationship to the outside world. In this way, each system within the person is motivated towards conditions of homoeostasis and aims to achieve, within limits, a certain constancy of function. Such ideas are not new, of course, and Roy acknowledges the impact that Helson's research into human adaptation had on the development of her nursing model. In particular, Helson's claims that all organisms strive to achieve optimum levels of *physiological* and *behavioural* homoeostasis has had particular influence on Roy's own work.

In his use of the first of these terms, Helson was referring to mechanisms that have as their effect the maintenance of relative balance in physiological systems such as those relating to fluid balance and the regulation of food intake. By the second, he was referring to tendencies that enable individuals to cope with new psychological or social experiences. Helson believed that, in much the same way as there are limits to the extent to which food and water can be satisfactorily ingested at any one time, there may be limits to the sorts of social experiences that a person can adequately deal with.

For both physiological and psychological systems there may, therefore, be said to exist conditions of relative equilibrium which a person aims to achieve. It is important to recognise, however, that these conditions must always be relative ones. The use of the term 'relative' in this context is intended to suggest that there exists a range of conditions of balance in which individuals are able to cope adequately with their environmental experience. There is no one absolute level of balance that people seek to attain.

It may be useful, therefore, to think of people as organisms concerned with maintaining their physiological and psychological systems within a range of conditions unique to themselves. According to Roy, such a set of conditions makes up a person's adaptation level, and new stimuli that fall within this range of possibilities are likely to be reacted to more favourably than those that fall outside

48

it. In one sense, therefore, a person's *adaptation level* is little more than a range of adaptability within which it is possible to deal adequately with new experiences. Such a situation is shown diagrammatically in Figure 6.1.

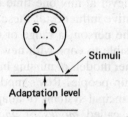

Stimuli

Adaptation level

Here can be seen stimuli falling outside the range of possibilities established by a person's adaptation level, thus leading to maladaptive and inefficient responses

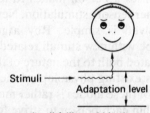

Stimuli

Adaptation level

Here can be seen stimuli falling within the range of possibilities established by a person's adaptation level, thus leading to effective coping responses

Figure 6.1   Adaptation level

Roy calls the factors influencing an individual's adaptation level *stimuli*, and further distinguishes between three types of these. The first, *focal stimuli*, are those immediately surrounding a person. In many nursing situations these may be those associated with the presence of nurses themselves and may include, for example, equipment and materials used to deliver nursing and clinical care. *Contextual stimuli*, on the other hand, are those that occur alongside focal stimuli. For example, if the delivery of nursing care takes place in an overly cold or unduly hot environment, such ambient temperatures may constitute contextual influences for other focal stimuli more directly impinging on the person. Finally *residual stimuli*, such as beliefs, attitudes and personal qualities, are

49

those resulting from past patterns of learning. For example, memories of earlier experiences in hospital can act as significant residual stimuli, combining with focal and contextual cues to affect a person's adaptation level.

An individual's adaptation level at any one time is, therefore, likely to be related to the relative influence of these three sets of stimuli, and establishes, for the person, a range of conditions of balance within which it is possible to cope with new experiences.

In much the same way as other models of nursing have identified a number of sub-systems within people, Roy's model of nursing argues that there exist four principal systems of adaptation influencing behaviour. These are called *modes of adaptation*, and they comprise the physiological, self-concept, role-function and interdependency systems.

The first of these modes of adaptation is very broad, encompassing the responses a person makes to temperature, food, fluids, oxygen and other sensory stimulation. Nevertheless, the underlying principle involved is simple. Roy argues that an individual's capacity to cope with new stimuli related to physiological needs is likely to be related both to the nature of the stimuli themselves and to the person's existing physiological mode of adaptation.

The second of these modes is rather more complex, and refers to tendencies within each person to strive for consistency in terms of self-understanding, both in terms of behaviour and in terms of relationships with others. This notion implies that there may be limits to the extent to which individuals can cope with changes in their bodily or psychological selves at any one time. It seems likely that such tendencies may have implications for the ways in which nurses prepare patients for surgical procedures which may result in a changed body image.

The third mode of adaptation highlights the possibility that tensions can arise when external demands on a person's role performance fall outside the range of roles to which adaptation is possible. For example, people who consider themselves to be reasonably active and fit may have difficulty in adapting to the more passive role that being in hospital sometimes requires.

The final mode of adaptation emphasises that individuals strive to attain conditions of relative balance in terms of relationships of friendliness, dominance and competitiveness. It alerts the nurse to the potential dangers that exist when people are presented with situations of dominance, aggression or familiarity outside their present levels of adaptation.

These four modes of adaptation and the consequences they have for the planning and delivery of nursing care are represented diagrammatically in Table 6.1.

Table 6.1   Four modes of adaptation

The person	Problems within mode of adaptation lead to
Physiological adaptive mode	Hyperactivity, fatigue Malnutrition, vomiting Constipation, incontinence Dehydration, oedema, electrolyte imbalance Oxygen deficit, oxygen excess Shock Fever, hypothermia Sensory deprivation, sensory overload Endocrine imbalance
Self-concept adaptive mode	Sense of physical loss Sense of guilt Sense of anxiety Sense of powerlessness Sense of social disengagement Sense of aggression
Role-function adaptive mode	Sense of role failure Sense of role conflict
Interdependency adaptive mode	Sense of alienation Sense of rejection Sense of rivalry Sense of loneliness Sense of dominance Sense of exhibition

The Causes of Problems Likely to Require Nursing Intervention

According to Roy, nursing interventions are likely to be necessary whenever there exists either a *need deficit* or a *need excess* within one or more of the four adaptive modes. By these terms is meant the existence of either an insufficiency of, or an excess within, the environmental resources available to a person, particular to one or more modes of adaptation.

The Nature of the Assessment Process

Given what has been said so far, nursing assessment using Roy's model of nursing will first of all seek to identify those modes within which adaptation problems exist. Such a first-stage assessment can be carried out relatively quickly, with the nurse using this model of nursing as a guide to aspects of behaviour which are particularly worthy of investigation. Using it, the nurse will examine in turn, patient adaptation within the physiological, self-concept, role-function and interdependency modes. Such a preliminary assessment, however, is likely to be followed by a second-stage and more detailed assessment, involving the identification of specific focal, contextual and residual stimuli relating to the adaptation problems identified. Reaching such diagnoses is likely to be dependent on the quality of the nurse–patient relationship and the extent to which the nurse encourages the patient to play an active role in the assessment process itself.

The Nature of the Planning and Goal-setting Process

In the light of findings from first- and second-stage assessments, the nurse is likely to draw up a list of goals relating to the patient concerned. These will need to be placed in an order of priority, and should be written in patient-centred terms. That is, they should specify what the patient should be able to do when the goal has been achieved. It may also be useful for the nurse to distinguish between short-term, intermediate and long-term nursing goals relating to each of the modes within which problems connected with adaptation have been identified.

The Focus of Intervention During the Implementation of the Care Plan

According to Roy's model, nursing interventions are likely to involve manipulating the relationship between environmental stimuli and the patient's adaptation level so that the former fall within the person's level of adaptation. This may be achieved in two distinct ways. First of all, the nurse may select, in delivering care, stimuli that fall within the patient's present range of adaptation, rejecting those that are likely to fall outside it. In so doing, the nurse may aim to maximise the familiarity that nursing interventions are likely to have for the patient, by restricting the use of technical language and nursing behaviours to those that the patient is likely to have experienced beforehand. Alternatively, the nurse may decide that it is the patient's present adaptation level that needs to be manipulated. This latter course of action may be decided upon when it is felt that aspects of necessary nursing and clinical care are likely to fall outside the patient's present range of adaptive responses.

The Nature of the Process of Evaluating the Quality and Effects of the Care Given

In terms of evaluating the effectiveness of nursing actions, the Roy model of nursing suggests that attention should be given to the extent to which maladaptation within each adaptive mode has been corrected as a result of interventions made. In doing this, the nurse will attempt to evaluate the success with which each goal has been accomplished.

The Role of the Nurse

Roy has described 'higher-level wellness' as the overall goal of the health-care team (Roy and Roberts, 1981). In working towards this broad goal, a distinction can be made between the role of doctors and that of nurses. Roy suggests that, while doctors focus on biological systems and disease processes, the nurse's specific role is to promote patient adaptation in health and illness. The role of the nurse, therefore, is primarily that of manipulating stimuli, especially focal stimuli, so that they come to fall within the patient's zone of adaptation.

Using Roy's Adaptation Model of Nursing with the Nursing Process

So far an attempt has been made to outline in general terms the concerns with which the Roy model of nursing works. It should also be apparent that, by using this model, nurses may be able to make their actions more systematic in assessing, planning, intervening in and evaluating nursing care. By looking at how such a model might be used in everyday nursing practice, it should be possible to clarify the usefulness of Roy's model of nursing for the planning and delivery of nursing care.

Assessment—First Stage

As has been pointed out, Roy suggests that the first stage of nursing assessment should be carried out fairly quickly. In doing this, nurses should aim to observe patient behaviour and from this decide whether or not there is a need for nursing intervention. For example, a teenage girl in hospital following the formation of an ileostomy may refuse to see any visitors, except her close family. The first stage of assessment might suggest to the nurse the existence of an adaptation problem in the self-concept mode. The nature of this will be further explored during the second stage of assessment. Similarly, a four-year-old child who has experienced many hospital admissions may show signs of aggression at the approach of the ward doctor. Here an initial assessment may suggest maladaptation within the interdependency adaptive mode, the child being unable to cope satisfactorily with this particular relationship.

Assessment—Second Stage

Having identified that there is some cause for concern in an individual's behaviour, the nurse moves to the second stage of

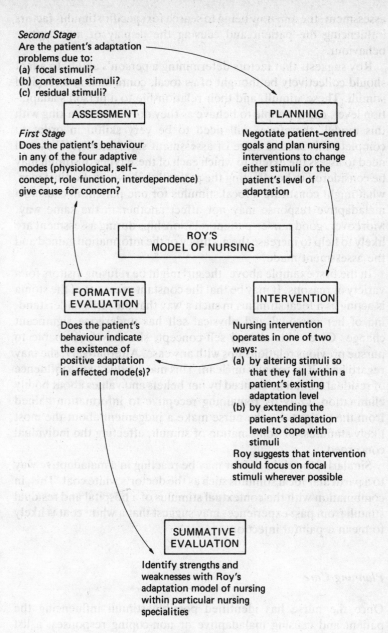

Second Stage
Are the patient's adaptation
problems due to:
(a) focal stimuli?
(b) contextual stimuli?
(c) residual stimuli?

ASSESSMENT

First Stage
Does the patient's behaviour
in any of the four adaptive
modes (physiological, self-
concept, role function, interdependence)
give cause for concern?

PLANNING

Negotiate patient-centred
goals and plan nursing
interventions to change
either stimuli or the
patient's level of
adaptation

ROY'S MODEL OF NURSING

FORMATIVE EVALUATION

Does the patient's
behaviour indicate
the existence of
positive adaptation
in affected mode(s)?

INTERVENTION

Nursing intervention
operates in one of two
ways:
(a) by altering stimuli so
that they fall within a
patient's existing
adaptation level
(b) by extending the
patient's adaptation
level to cope with
stimuli
Roy suggests that intervention
should focus on focal
stimuli wherever possible

SUMMATIVE EVALUATION

Identify strengths and
weaknesses with Roy's
adaptation model of nursing
within particular nursing
specialities

Figure 6.2

55

assessment, the aim now being to search for specific stimulus factors influencing the patient and causing the display of maladaptive behaviour.

Roy suggests that factors determining a person's ability to adapt should collectively be thought of as focal, contextual and residual stimuli. These stimuli, and their relationship to a person's adaptation level, cause people to behave as they do. Nurses working with this model, therefore, will need to be very skilful in order to complete this second stage of assessment satisfactorily. They will need to assess the extent to which each of these types of stimuli may be considered to be affecting the patient's behaviour. For instance, what might constitute a focal stimulus for one patient in causing a maladaptive response may not affect another in the same way. Moreover, good nurse–patient relationships during assessment are likely to help to increase the accuracy of the information gained and the assessment made.

In the first example above, the girl might be refusing visitors for a variety of reasons. It may be that the constant presence of the stoma is acting as a focal stimulus in such a way that the girl's understanding of her personal and physical self has undergone significant change. Given this altered self-concept, she may feel unable to pursue previous relationships with any ease. Alternatively, she may regard herself as socially unclean. This may be due to the influence of residual stimuli influenced by her beliefs and values about bodily elimination. Only by remaining receptive to information gained from the patient can the nurse make a judgement about the most likely stimulus, or combination of stimuli, affecting the individual concerned.

Similarly, the child of four may be reacting in a maladaptive way to a particular focal stimulus such as the doctor's white coat. This, in combination with the contextual stimulus of a hospital and residual stimuli from past experience, may suggest that a white coat is likely to mean a painful injection.

Planning Care

Once the nurse has identified possible stimuli influencing the patient and causing maladaptive or non-coping responses, a list should be made of the goals that it is hoped the patient will be able

56

to achieve. Roy sees the long-term goals of nursing care as enabling patients to adapt positively to, or cope effectively with, an ever-changing environment.

In the short-term, however, goals set are likely to be those specifying an extended adaptation level in one or more modes of adaptation.

To return to the two examples, an intermediate goal for the teenage girl might be that she feels able to spend time with a number of friends during visiting time. To achieve this, some short-term goals might be set relating to the girl's renewed acceptance of her personal and physical self. If detailed observation has led the nurse to believe that the child of four is behaving aggressively to the stimulus of a white coat, then plans may be made either to alter this stimulus or to help the child to adapt more positively towards it.

Nursing Intervention and the Delivery of Care

Roy's model of nursing suggests that every person strives to attain a state of relative physiological and psychological equilibrium. Nursing intervention, therefore, aims either to effect a change in the relevant stimuli affecting a person so that these fall within the individual's adaptation level, or to change their adaptation level so as to enable the individual to cope more effectively with them.

Returning to the examples may help to clarify the nursing actions likely to be involved in the care of these two patients. Roy suggests that, whenever possible, the nurse should manipulate focal stimuli first of all, since these are most likely to be the primary causes of the patient's behaviour.

While it will not be possible for the nurse to remove the focal stimulus of the stoma for the teenage girl, it may be possible to extend her adaptation level by introducing her to another young person who has successfully adapted to the formation of a stoma.

With the child of four, the nurse may first aim to effect change in the relationship between the focal stimulus of the white coat and the child's ability to cope with it. One possible intervention might be to ask the doctor to avoid wearing the coat concerned. Alternatively, the nurse might intervene to extend the child's adaptation level by introducing him to games that involve play with, or dressing up in, a white coat.

57

Successful evaluation of any nursing intervention can only take place if goals have first been set. These should indicate the patient-behaviours that the nurse will expect following successful nursing intervention. Thus, in planning care with Roy's model of nursing, nurses should aim to identify behaviours in particular adaptive modes that will indicate when goals have been met.

So, in evaluating the nursing care given to the teenage girl, the nurse is likely to look for evidence of positive adaptation in the self-concept mode, and, in time, the girl may be prepared to receive more visitors and may verbally express more positive views about her personal and physical self.

Similarly, in evaluating the care planned for the child of four, the nurse might expect to observe more friendly behaviour towards the doctor, indicating the presence of a more adaptive response within the interdependency mode.

It should be stressed, however, that formative evaluation should be carried out continuously throughout the delivery of care, and may not always indicate that successful nursing intervention has taken place. Formative evaluation and reassessment are therefore closely linked within the application of this model of nursing.

For the Roy adaptation model to prove credible to practising nurses, it needs careful evaluation over time. To achieve this summative evaluation, practising nurses and nurse managers need to be willing to implement the model in a variety of nursing contexts and to evaluate its overall usefulness as a set of guidelines for planning and delivering care.

7

Orem's Self-Care Model of Nursing

Introduction

Like the models of nursing developed by Johnson (1980) and Roy (1980), Orem's Self-Care model emphasises the existence of biological, psychological and social systems within the person. Butterfield (1983), however, has argued that Orem's model of nursing differs from these other models in terms of its commitment to the concept of the person as a whole.

Before the model is examined in detail, the concept of Self-Care, around which Orem has based her model of nursing, needs to be explained. Orem (1985) defines Self-Care as '. . . the practice of activities that individuals initiate and perform on their own behalf in maintaining life, health and well-being . . .'. Thus, Self-Care is a concept applicable to individuals when they are in a state of health and well-being, rather than when they are in a state of ill-health or sickness. While it must be acknowledged that some nurses have expressed doubts about whether an absolute level of well-being can ever exist, by focusing on an individual's state of health, Orem's model of nursing takes a distinctive stance as an approach to care. This model of nursing, therefore, is one that emphasises activities that maintain life, health and well-being. It is also a model that values personal responsibility for health, while recognising that prevention and health education can be key aspects of nursing intervention.

In her writing, Orem (1980, 1985) suggests that western society

59

expects adults to be self-reliant and to take a degree of personal responsibility for their dependants. Such a view accords to some extent with those expressed by writers such as Illich (1976) in their critique of the increasing medicalisation of everyday life, and in analysing people's increasing reliance on hospital care.

As with other models, Orem's model of nursing will be examined more closely in terms of what it has to say about seven core aspects of people and their nursing care.

Key Components of Care

The Nature of People

According to Orem, a person is a functional, integrated whole with a motivation to achieve Self-Care. Individuals constantly act to maintain a balance between their abilities to achieve Self-Care and the various demands that are made on their *Self-Care Abilities*. This idea—that people strive to maintain a state of both bodily and psychological equilibrium—is, in many ways, a familiar one. Both Johnson and Roy, in their models of nursing, have argued for the existence of such homoeostatic tendencies in people. However, the notion of balance implied by Orem's model is somewhat different from a more conventional approach to understanding homo-eostasis, since, in this nursing model, the emphasis is on the maintenance of balance between a person's ability to act to achieve Self-Care and the various demands made on this ability. This balance should be considered important regardless of whether a person is in a state of health or ill-health. However, for a healthy individual, Orem identifies eight *Universal Self-Care Needs* that require satisfaction (Table 7.1).

A healthy person is likely to have sufficient Self-Care Abilities to meet these fundamental needs. Such a situation can be represented diagrammatically as in Figure 7.1. However, an individual who has experienced injury, disease or illness is likely to have additional demands for Self-Care. Orem calls these demands *Health Deviation Self-Care Needs*. Three types of these are singled out for particular attention: those related to changes in a person's physical *structure*; to changes in physical *function*; and to changes in *behaviour*.

60

Table 7.1   Orem's Universal Self-Care needs

(1) Sufficient intake of air
(2) Sufficient intake of water
(3) Sufficient intake of food
(4) Satisfactory eliminative functions
(5) Activity balanced with rest
(6) Time spent alone balanced with time spent with others
(7) Prevention of danger to the self
(8) Being 'normal'

A change in physical structure might follow a skin burn or could take the form of a local swelling resulting from a sting. A change in physical functioning might accompany a severely strained ankle or might follow childbirth, with the production of breast milk. Behavioural changes could include alterations in eating habits or difficulties associated with sleeping.

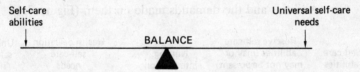

Figure 7.1   A healthy individual

If a person is able to meet these additional demands for Self-Care from existing Self-Care Abilities, then overall balance is likely to be maintained and nursing will not be required (Figure 7.2).

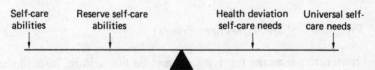

Figure 7.2   An individual subject to injury, disease or illness

The Causes of Problems Likely to Require Nursing Intervention

For those working with the Orem model of nursing, nursing intervention is indicated only when individuals (or their relatives and significant others) are unable to achieve or maintain a balance between their Self-Care Abilities and the demands made on these. Such a situation will occur when Self-Care Demands exceed the Self-Care Abilities of a particular person (Figure 7.3).

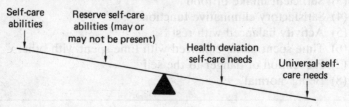

Figure 7.3 An individual in need of nursing intervention

According to Orem, the need for nursing arises from health-related experiences. In other words, adults will not normally require nursing to meet their Universal Self-Care Needs unless there are also Health Deviation Self-Care Needs affecting them. Thus, nursing interventions aim to restore a balance between Self-Care Abilities and the demands made on them (Figure 7.4).

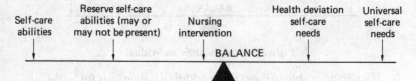

Figure 7.4 An individual in receipt of nursing intervention

The Nature of the Assessment Process

Orem rarely uses the term 'assessment' in her writing. Instead she talks of nurses undertaking an *investigative operation* to arrive at a nursing diagnosis. However, her professed commitment to the use of the nursing process allows us to regard an investigative operation as synonymous with assessment.

Orem suggests that, by seeking five types of information from patients, nurses will be able to make decisions about the planning and implementation of care.

First of all, the nurse needs to assess those demands being made on the individual for Self-Care. Second, an assessment must be made of the individual's ability to meet these demands. These two processes, taken together, form the first stage of the assessment procedure, and following this a decision can be made about the need for nursing intervention.

Third, if a Self-Care deficit is found to exist, the nurse must establish the reasons for it. Orem suggests a number of possible areas for further assessment in connection with identifying such causes. One reason a deficit exists may be because the individual possesses insufficient *knowledge* to respond to Self-Care Demands. Alternatively, a person may have insufficient *skill* to be able to carry out necessary Self-Care Activities. *Motivation* to achieve Self-Care is also important, as is the individual's *stage of development* and *past experience*. The influence of this last factor may be to limit the person's scope for Self-Care to behaviours and roles thought to be culturally acceptable. There is some similarity between such a notion and Johnson's (1980) emphasis on choice as a structural element in each of the behavioural sub-systems postulated by her model of nursing.

Fourth, the nurse must assess whether the individual's present state allows for safe involvement in Self-Care.

Finally, nurses need to assess the patient's potential for re-establishing Self-Care in the future.

As has been seen with previous nursing models, the process of assessment should be neither haphazard nor intuitive. Orem argues that, if patients are adequately assessed, these five kinds of information should provide sufficient qualitative and quantitative data on which to make decisions about nursing interventions. While acknowledging that patients differ from one another in terms of their overall needs, Orem advocates the gathering of information about these five key areas for every individual.

Two additional factors are worthy of note. Orem sees assessment as a continuous process, with more information being gathered as the relationship develops between nurse and patient. She also argues for the involvement of the individual's family and significant others in the assessment process, since her model of nursing emphasises not only the value of Self-Care, but also the value of caring for dependents.

The Nature of the Planning and Goal-setting Process

Although Orem does not explicitly argue for it, it is advocated that, as before, all goals should be patient-centred. It is further suggested that occasions will arise when it is appropriate to set short-term, intermediate and long-term goals, or specific combinations of these.

A significant emphasis in this model of nursing, however, requires the nurse to negotiate with the patient at the planning stage, whether nursing intervention is to be *wholly compensatory*, *partly compensatory* or *supportive-educative*. Thus, in preparing a patient for Self-Care, the nurse can act for the patient completely, share certain tasks with the patient or intervene in a way that is broadly consultative and facilitative.

The Focus of Intervention During the Implementation of the Care Plan

Implementing the care plan is likely to involve both nurse and patient in activities to help to meet Self-Care Demands. In addition, members of the patient's family and significant others may also provide care. Orem has identified six broad ways in which nurses can assist in implementing a care plan (Table 7.2). It should be remembered, however, that each of these methods of helping requires a complementary role from the patient. For example, if the nurse is acting for the patient, the latter must be prepared to be the recipient of that care. Indeed, Orem's model assumes both that patients are willing and able to adopt certain roles and that they desire to achieve Self-Care.

Table 7.2   Ways in which a care plan may be implemented

---

(1) Doing for or acting for another
(2) Guiding or directing another
(3) Providing physical support
(4) Providing psychological support
(5) Providing an environment which supports development
(6) Teaching another

The Nature of the Process of Evaluating the Quality and Effects of the Care Given

Orem suggests that nurses should evaluate care in terms of the patient's or family's subsequent ability to perform Self-Care. To measure this, at specified times each goal originally set must be considered to identify the extent to which it has been achieved. More generally, a move from nursing intervention that is wholly compensatory to that which seeks to support patients in the performance of Self-Care should be taken as a sign of effective nursing intervention.

A patient's success in maintaining a balance between Self-Care Demands and Self-Care Abilities is likely to depend both on an increased capacity to perform Self-Care Activities and on alterations in Self-Care Demands. Orem calls the latter type of change *recovery*—a term she uses in a broadly similar way to its more general use in the medical model of care.

The Role of the Nurse

According to Orem, the nurse's major role is a complementary one related to the individual's need and ability to undertake Self-Care. Nurses may intervene in the lives of their patients in order to help the individual to sustain health, recover from disease and injury or cope with the effects of disease and injury. Orem also acknowledges that nurses have a more particular role to play when specialised care is required.

Using Orem's Self-Care Model with the Nursing Process

Orem's Self-Care model of nursing encourages nurses to act in a complementary way with patients, their families and significant others in order to enable Self-Care to be achieved. Orem believes that, for each person, whether in health or ill-health, there is a balance between the ability to carry out Self-Care and demands made on this. Nursing intervention is required when, for whatever reason, this balance is upset. Primarily, the reason for imbalance is

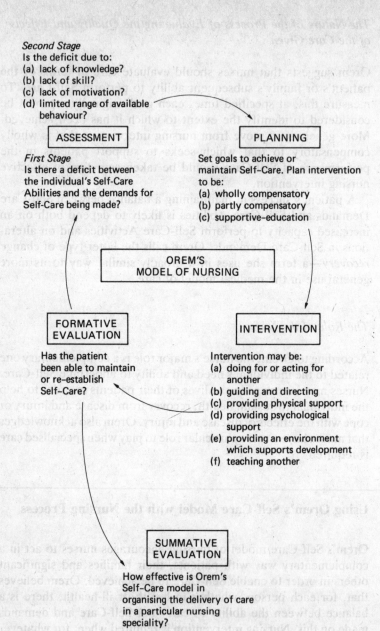

Second Stage
Is the deficit due to:
(a) lack of knowledge?
(b) lack of skill?
(c) lack of motivation?
(d) limited range of available behaviour?

ASSESSMENT

First Stage
Is there a deficit between the individual's Self-Care Abilities and the demands for Self-Care being made?

PLANNING

Set goals to achieve or maintain Self-Care. Plan intervention to be:
(a) wholly compensatory
(b) partly compensatory
(c) supportive–education

OREM'S MODEL OF NURSING

FORMATIVE EVALUATION

Has the patient been able to maintain or re-establish Self-Care?

INTERVENTION

Intervention may be:
(a) doing for or acting for another
(b) guiding and directing
(c) providing physical support
(d) providing psychological support
(e) providing an environment which supports development
(f) teaching another

SUMMATIVE EVALUATION

How effective is Orem's Self-Care model in organising the delivery of care in a particular nursing speciality?

Figure 7.5

66

likely to be injury, disease or illness, all of which imply the existence of Health Deviation Self-Care Needs which the patient may, or may not, be able to meet. By briefly considering how the model might be implemented with the nursing process, a better understanding of it is likely to develop.

Assessment—First Stage

The first stage of the process of assessment aims to determine whether or not a need for nursing intervention exists. Nurses working with Orem's model, therefore, are likely to identify individuals' demands for Self-Care and their present abilities to meet these. For example, in carrying out an initial assessment of a young man in a leg plaster following a road accident, who is unable to move around unaided, it is likely that the nurse will identify an imbalance between his ability to carry out Self-Care and the demands for Self-Care made on him. Similarly, a mother may experience difficulty in meeting the demands made on her by her young daughter when the latter is suffering from one of the common childhood infectious diseases. Here there exists an imbalance between the mother's Self-Care Abilities that can be used to assist in the care of others and demands currently being made on these.

Assessment—Second Stage

It having been decided that nursing intervention is required, the next stage of the assessment process involves the gathering of information to decide why there is a Self-Care Deficit. By observation and discussion, the nurse should be able to link the Self-Care Deficit to a lack of knowledge or skills, to a lack of motivation to achieve Self-Care or, perhaps, to behaviours limited by social and cultural norms.

In the first example above, it is likely that the young man will need to learn some new skills to cope with his present situation in order to re-establish his capacity for Self-Care. In the second example, the mother may lack knowledge of the kind of behaviour she is likely to witness in her daughter while the latter experiences, perhaps, a high temperature or skin discomfort. She may also be

67

poorly motivated to care for her daughter if she lacks confidence in her ability to extend her own Self-Care capacities to others.

Planning Care

Once the nurse has identified reasons for a patient's Self-Care Deficit, it is possible for patient-centred goals to be set and for intervention to be planned. With Orem's model of nursing, the long-term goal for each patient is likely to be the restoration of balance between Self-Care Abilities and Self-Care Needs. The extent to which nursing intervention will take place depends on the extent to which Self-Care can be undertaken by patients, their families and significant others.

Thus, in the first example, planned nursing interventions are likely to be both partly compensatory and supportive-educative. The young man is likely to be able to meet Universal Self-Care Demands such as eating and drinking, by himself. However, the nurse may plan to aid his mobility in the short term, and may plan also to help him learn new skills by which to avoid a recurrence of the accident which resulted in hospitalisation in the first place. In the second example, the nurse may plan to intervene in a way which is supportive-educative, so that the mother can care for her dependent daughter during the child's illness.

Nursing Intervention and the Delivery of Care

As already described, nurses have a number of methods of intervention open to them. The aim of intervention in each case, however, will be to help each patient to maintain or re-establish Self-Care.

Initially, the young man in a leg plaster may require that certain tasks be carried out for him by the nurse. These might include the putting on and taking off of trousers. In this instance, the nurse is likely to be acting for the patient. The nurse may also teach the patient new skills, so that, with time, he can accomplish more of his care for himself. For example, instruction might be given in how greater use of the arms can facilitate movement from bed to chair.

68

The nurse may also arrange a suitable environment in which the patient feels able to develop these new skills.

To assist the mother in caring for her daughter, the nurse may teach her about the usual course of a particular childhood complaint and may instruct her in ways of making the child more comfortable. The mother may also be helped by the nurse's provision of psychological support in the form of positive reinforcement. This could be achieved by praising actions taken by the mother which indicate a more confident and safe approach to the care of the child.

Evaluation

Orem's Self-Care model of nursing clearly emphasises a commitment to the value of Self-Care. Thus, formative evaluation is likely to focus on the extent to which the balance between Self-Care Abilities and Self-Care Demands has been maintained or re-established. By setting goals that are patient-centred, nurses put themselves in a position to evaluate *what patients have achieved* at the end of specified periods of time, rather than whether or not nursing intervention has been carried out.

Thus, in formatively evaluating the nursing care planned and delivered for the young man, the nurse is likely to look for evidence in his behaviour to show an increasing ability to undertake Self-Care. By doing this, the nurse may find, for example, that the frequency of nursing interventions involving acting for the patient may decrease with time. Similarly, a move from nursing interventions that are wholly or partly compensatory to those that are broadly supportive-educative in nature would also indicate effective nursing care.

With respect to formatively evaluating the success of nursing interventions encouraging the mother's attempts to care for the child, her verbal expression of greater confidence and an ability to carry out appropriate care may, with time, obviate the need for nursing intervention at all.

Finally, in summatively evaluating Orem's model, nurses are likely to explore its usefulness in planning and delivering care across a range of settings and with a variety of patients. By doing this, it may be possible to identify nursing contexts in which the model seems particularly useful. Additionally, before a decision is made about whether to work with Orem's model of nursing, practising nurses may need to spend some time considering whether the concept of the patient, the role of the nurse and the values with which the model works are in accordance with those which they hold to be true to good nursing practice today.

8

Riehl's Interactionist
Model of Nursing

Introduction

The models of nursing so far described offer nurses a variety of
approaches to the planning and delivery of patient care. However,
to a greater or lesser extent, they have certain features in common,
in that they emphasise the existence of bodily, psychological and
social systems within people which influence behaviour. In recent
years a number of nurses have begun to criticise models such as
these for being too mechanistic in their identification of human
needs. It has been argued, for example, that drawing an analogy
between a human being and a machine with parts and systems
within it, is likely to dehumanise the process of nursing itself.
Instead such critics have argued for the development of nursing
models which take as their starting point the human ability to reason
and act in ways that are *meaningful*.

According to this alternative perspective, people behave as they
do, not because of the workings of systems within them, but because
of meanings attached to the actions they perform. Should such ideas
be made a central focus in a nursing model, it is argued, nursing
might be able to move some way towards establishing itself as a set
of practices with some autonomy from those of other health-care
professions, many of which operate with somewhat mechanistic
conceptions of people and their health-related needs.

To argue that a shift of attention away from an examination of
systems within the person to one focusing on how people make

sense of their immediate experiences is not to claim that an understanding of physiological processes would thereby become entirely irrelevant to nursing. These would always remain as one focus of nursing interest, since they often have consequences for the ways in which people function psychologically and socially. However, by emphasising the importance of processes by which patients come to make sense of behaviour in what are often unfamiliar surroundings, a model of nursing could take a radical stance compared with more conventional approaches to care.

An emphasis on human beings as *givers of meaning* to the situations they encounter is at one with an approach to explaining human behaviour developed by a group of social scientists called the *symbolic interactionists*. One of them, Mead (1934), believed that an important human quality is that associated with the capacity to understand the world in terms of symbols. By the term 'symbol' is meant a word, image or action that stands for something else. Humans spend much of their time communicating with one another (or failing to do so) via symbols. Hence, the term 'symbolic interactionist' is used to identify someone who is particularly interested in analysing the ways in which symbolic communication takes place.

Early in his work, Mead noticed that meanings attached to symbols appear to be widely shared within a culture. For example, within the culture of car drivers, the symbols shown in Figure 8.1 have relatively clear meanings associated with them. However, there are not many symbols whose meanings are universally clear and unambiguous. Thus, while the meanings attached to particular symbols are often understood by others, they are unlikely to be universally shared by all. In nursing, too, there exist many symbols, some of which will be familiar to those who come into regular contact with them (Figure 8.2). However, showing symbols such as these to nurses other than those working in Britain would, perhaps, reveal that, even within the nursing community, the meanings that particular symbols have vary enormously.

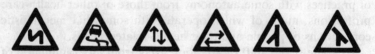

Figure 8.1   Symbols with relatively clear meanings

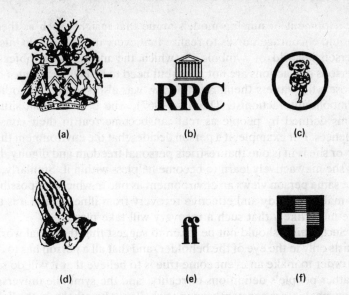

(a)   (b)   (c)

(d)   (e)   (f)

Figure 8.2   Symbols used in the nursing press: (a) The Royal Marsden Hospital; (b) the Rapid Results College; (c) Lincolnshire County Council; (d) St Oswald's Hospice, Newcastle upon Tyne; (e) Faber and Faber; (f) Nuffield Hospitals. Taken from advertisements in *Nursing Times*, October 1985

It seems reasonable to suggest, therefore, that a hospital environment, full of equipment, apparatus and notices that may have meaning for nursing staff, can appear frightening to those who do not normally work in such settings. If qualified nurses working in routine ward environments sometimes find the technical equipment of the intensive care unit unfamiliar and threatening, then it may be salutary to pause for a moment to imagine how this situation might appear to patients.

According to symbolic interactionists, when individuals are confronted with unfamiliar situations, they try to 'make sense' of them as best they can by drawing on past experience. Hence, patients and nurses unfamiliar with a high-technology area in a care setting may liken it to a set from a science fiction film. Similarly, because of past experiences and expectations, a dimly lit and unkempt day-area in a ward for the elderly may be perceived by those nursed within it as resembling a Dickensian work-house.

Those who advocate the use of symbolic interactionist ideas in the development of nursing models argue that insights such as these should encourage nurses to realise that every individual inhabits a personal world of symbols, in which the meanings of objects, persons and actions are not given but need to be *actively created* by those who witness them. Such a view was also shared by another symbolic interactionist, Thomas (1967), who believed that situations defined by people as real can become real in their consequences. For example, if a person decides that the environment that he or she is in is one that restricts personal freedom and dignity, he or she may actively learn to become helpless within it. Similarly, if the same person views an environment as one in which it is possible to make a speedy and effective recovery from illness, then it is all the more likely that such a recovery will take place.

Such claims should not be taken to suggest that the social world exists only in the eye of the beholder, and that all a person has to do in order to make an event come true is to believe that it will do so. Rather people's definitions of reality, and the symbolic universes they inhabit, are constantly open to challenge by others. In the light of this, symbolic interactionists talk about social situations being *negotiated* between those present. Through such negotiation, definitions of particular situations arise which are the outcome of processes in which different accounts of the same reality are tested against one another.

As an example of how nurses and patients might become involved in such a process of negotiation, it may be interesting to consider the case of the patient who insists on undertaking everyday office work in the ward after being admitted for an operation. In such a situation the nurses may be concerned that the individual involved changes his or her behaviour and attitudes to become more like other patients about to receive similar forms of care. If this is so, the nurse's expectations of what is reasonable behaviour in the ward may come into conflict with those of the patient, who may still see himself or herself as at work. The successful care of such a patient is likely to require a degree of mutual accommodation between these conflicting versions of reality, with the patient and nurse re-negotiating an acceptable solution intermediate between these two extremes.

From this background of symbolic interactionist thought, it may be possible to develop nursing models, and Riehl's (1980) interactionist model of nursing is one such approach to patient care. As with other models, it will be examined in detail by looking at what it has to say about seven core aspects of people and nursing care. Then an attempt will be made to explore how such a model might be applied using the nursing process.

Key Components of Care

The Nature of People

Riehl's model of nursing, in working with a number of insights derived from symbolic interactionist theory, argues that those receiving nursing care are individuals constantly striving to make sense of the situations they find themselves in. It further suggests that people are likely to differ from one another in terms of the ways in which they 'make sense' of the same situation.

Part of the nurse's role, therefore, involves an attempt to enter into the subjective world of patients in order to see things as they do. Only by doing this can a nurse make an accurate assessment of an individual's needs and plan an appropriate series of nursing interventions.

The Causes of Problems Likely to Require Nursing Intervention

Riehl argues that nursing problems arise when there are disturbances within one or more major aspects of a patient's behaviour. She calls these aspects *parameters:* the physiological, psychological and sociological parameters. Disturbance within any one of these is likely to have consequences both for itself and for the workings of other parameters. For example, changes within the psychological parameter brought on by being in the novel environment of a hospital or health centre can have implications for physiological processes, such as those associated with stress and reactions to it.

However, while Riehl argues that it is useful to see the origins of nursing problems in terms of disturbances associated with one or more of these three factors, her model of nursing is one which emphasises the importance of psychological and sociological parameters as critical determinants of human behaviour. Her model of

75

nursing therefore, differs from others so far described, in that it seeks to underplay the importance of physiological processes as causes of patient problems.

The Nature of the Assessment Process

Riehl seems keen to see nurses using a systematic approach to the assessment of patient needs. In her early work, she mentioned with approval the FANCAP system of assessment developed by Abbey (1980). This is a mnemonic device which nurses can use to assess patient needs within six areas of human activity important for 'the maintenance of a live, interacting, pain-free person' (Figure 8.3). More recently, however, Riehl (1985) had begun work on devising as assessment tool for specific use with this model of nursing.

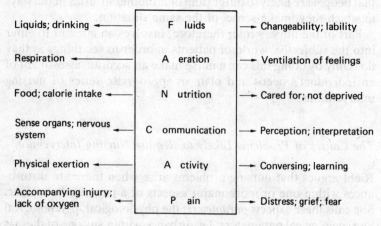

Figure 8.3 FANCAP—a system for the assessment of patient and client needs. Nurses assess each of the six aspects of patients specified by the mnemonic FANCAP, paying particular attention to the range of functions covered by each of these

Using either of these techniques, nurses are likely in the first stage of assessment to try to ascertain whether there is a need for nursing intervention. Having reached the conclusion that there is, a second stage of assessment may follow in which nurses will try to gain insight into patients' subjective perceptions of problems affecting them. After this an attempt is likely to be made to find out what *roles* have been previously adopted in coping with problems similar to these. By doing this nurses will be attempting to gain both an *intersubjective understanding* of the ways in which patients see their situation and an assessment of the *role performances* that are available to them as coping responses to these. An effective second-stage assessment should make it possible to determine the degree of role flexibility open to a particular patient and will allow the nurse to anticipate problems that might later arise when encouraging the development of new roles.

The Nature of the Planning and Goal-setting Process

Given that the focus of nursing care using Riehl's model of nursing is likely to be on the development of a relationship between nurse and patient, the use of short-term goals will be of considerable value. Their use is likely to allow care planning to remain sensitive to patients' changing needs and to nurses' increased understanding of patients' perceptions. Therefore, goals set will be a product of processes of negotiation between patient and nurse. Riehl suggests that goals should be written in patient-centred terms and should be identified for each problem anticipated from the assessment of the patient.

The Focus of Intervention During the Implementation of the Care Plan

For nurses working with Riehl's model, the majority of nursing interventions are likely to focus on the need to help patients to develop role flexibility to cope with their new status as people in receipt of nursing (and other) care. Some of the new roles that a person is likely to need to acquire will be connected with their medical status. Others may be related to the likely effects of hospitalisation or the special demands that nursing care imposes on an individual.

At this stage of nursing care it is likely that the nurse will be involved in *role-taking* with patients. In her writing, Riehl draws a distinction between this and *role play*—a contrast developed from the work of Coutu (1951). Whereas the latter is likely to involve both mental activity and changes in observable behaviour, role-taking primarily involves thinking about a situation from another's point of view. By encouraging patients to involve themselves in role-taking, the nurse will be hoping to achieve three goals. First, an attempt will be made to attain further degrees of intersubjective insight into patients' perceptions and needs. Second, efforts will be made to encourage patients to perceive their present situation in alternative ways. Third, by involving patients in activities requiring them to take the roles of others, nurses hope to encourage them to explore alternative roles that can be adopted in particular situations.

The Nature of the Process of Evaluating the Quality and Effects of the Care Given

According to Riehl's model of nursing, evaluation is likely to take place through an examination of the extent to which patients have acquired or developed new role performances that enable them to cope more adequately with problems identified. An initial formative evaluation of this type having been carried out, there may then be a subsequent need to re-assess patient needs and plan future care.

Summative evaluation of Riehl's model of nursing, on the other hand, is likely to require nurses to explore the effectiveness of this particular nursing model compared with others based upon insights from symbolic interactionist theory, such as those of Travelbee (1966) or of Duldt and Giffin (1985), in planning and delivering care across a variety of nursing situations.

The Role of the Nurse

Within Riehl's model of nursing, it is repeatedly emphasised that nurses should involve themselves as fully as possible in the subjective worlds of their patients. Only by doing this will it be possible to arrive at an accurate assessment of individual needs. Furthermore, the use of role-taking as a primary mode of nursing intervention would seem to suggest that the role of the nurse should aim to complement that of the patient. Thus, nurses working with

78

Riehl's model of nursing should aim to be empathetic and supportive towards their patients, while at the same time recognising that the patient–nurse relationship is best established within a framework of trust and equality.

Using Riehl's Model of Nursing with the Nursing Process

The preceding description of Riehl's model of nursing has emphasised the need for nurses to try to enter into the subjective worlds of their patients in applying this model in clinical practice. A number of suggestions will now be made about how, more specifically, this model of nursing might be applied using the nursing process.

Assessment—First Stage

As with most models of nursing, the first stage of assessment aims to determine whether or not the patient is in need of nursing intervention. In the case of nurses working with Riehl's model, a first-stage assessment is likely to involve making judgements about the appropriateness of the roles the patient adopts in different situations. Thus, a midwife working in an antenatal clinic might identify a pregnant woman as being in need of nursing intervention should she express serious doubts about her ability to care for her baby immediately after birth. Similarly, a nurse working in an acute trauma unit might assess a teenager refusing medication while in pain following a rib injury as in need of nursing intervention.

Having identified a need for nursing intervention in both these instances, the nurse working with Riehl's model of nursing would begin the second stage of assessment with a view to developing a better understanding of the role the patient is adopting and the causes of this.

Assessment—Second Stage

While this model of nursing is not a systems model of nursing in the way that others described earlier have been, Riehl nevertheless

79

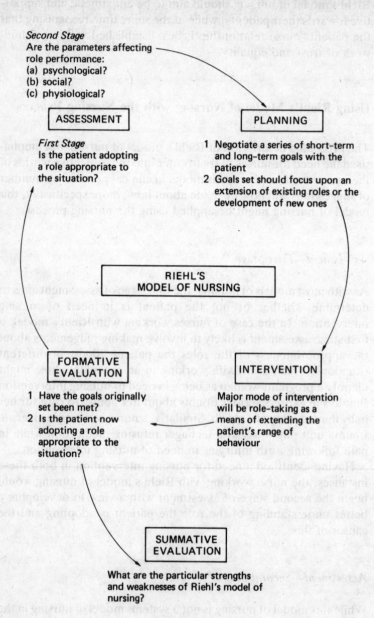

Second Stage
Are the parameters affecting
role performance:
(a) psychological?
(b) social?
(c) physiological?

ASSESSMENT

First Stage
Is the patient adopting
a role appropriate to
the situation?

PLANNING

1 Negotiate a series of short-term
  and long-term goals with the
  patient
2 Goals set should focus upon an
  extension of existing roles or the
  development of new ones

RIEHL'S
MODEL OF NURSING

FORMATIVE
EVALUATION

1 Have the goals originally
  set been met?
2 Is the patient now
  adopting a role
  appropriate to the
  situation?

INTERVENTION

Major mode of intervention
will be role-taking as a
means of extending the
patient's range of
behaviour

SUMMATIVE
EVALUATION

What are the particular strengths
and weaknesses of Riehl's model of
nursing?

Figure 8.4

advocates the use of a *systematic* approach to patient assessment. For this reason, the use of an assessment tool such as FANCAP may seem appropriate in exploring the nature of physiological, psychological and sociological parameters having an effect upon the patient.

Thus, the midwife assessing the mother-to-be might discover that, after the child's birth, considerable constraint may be placed on the woman's freedom to leave her home with the baby, because of its location and distance from public amenities and transport. In such circumstances, it might be decided that a problem within the sociological parameter is inhibiting the woman's ability to prepare for her new role performances following the birth of her child.

In carrying out a second-stage assessment of the teenager refusing medication for chest pain, the nurse should bear in mind that his present role performance is likely to increase the chances of his developing a chest infection due to shallowness of breathing. It might further be decided that such behaviour is likely to be caused by factors associated with both physiological and psychological parameters. In order to plan care for such an individual, however, it will be necessary for the nurse to gain a more complete appreciation of factors influencing the teenager's refusal of pain relief. This is likely to be achieved by a more thorough exploration of how he at present perceives himself and the care he is receiving.

Throughout both stages of assessment, however, the nurse should remember that the main purpose of this is to gain a better understanding of the patient's actions from the *patient's own* point of view.

Planning Care

Having gained information during assessment enabling patient problems to be related to particular parameters affecting behaviour, the nurse should negotiate with the patient a series of short-term and long-term goals. In view of the fact that Riehl's model underplays a traditional emphasis on restoring balance in physiological systems, goals should be patient-centred and *behavioural* in nature.

Thus, as an outcome of the midwife's negotiations with the mother-to-be, it may be decided that as a long-term goal the patient

81

will express positive attitudes about her ability to cope with the new baby. Along the way to achieving this, however, a number of short-term goals may be set, and, in working towards these, opportunities should arise for nurse and patient to develop their abilities to interpret each other's actions more accurately.

Similarly, the nurse concerned with the care of the teenager refusing medication for pain relief may negotiate as a long-term goal that he will be pain-free. However, more immediate goals may involve his adopting a different role with respect to receiving medication.

Nursing Intervention and the Delivery of Care

After gaining a better understanding of how patients see the situations they are in, nurses put themselves in the position of being able to intervene to extend the range of roles open to those in their care. It is hoped that doing this will enable patients to acquire new roles, or develop existing ones, to enable them to cope more adequately in situations requiring nursing care. One of the most effective ways of extending the range of roles that a person can adopt is through role-taking and possibly role play.

Thus, the midwife may try to consider the difficulties facing the pregnant woman to help her understand the situation from the patient's point of view. By doing this, the midwife may be able to begin to appreciate that the demands of motherhood in this case are likely to be particularly taxing, given the patient's circumstances. Additionally, the pregnant woman might be encouraged to imagine situations likely to arise after the birth of her child. By so doing, she may think of ways to cope with situations previously thought impossible. As a result of this role-taking, some accommodation between the expectations of the midwife and the patient may take place. This may lead to some compromise being reached between the style of child care the midwife finds acceptable and that which the mother originally felt she could manage.

Similarly, some role-taking between himself and other members of the health-care team might help the teenager to adopt a more appropriate role relating to his injury. It could also result in a modification of the nurse's view of the patient. In order to help him to see the situation from another perspective, the nurse might encourage the teenager to think about the role of the physiotherapist involved in his care. Concurrent with this, the nurse might try to imagine the situation from the patient's point of view, which may make it possible to learn more about the reasons underlying the teenager's refusal of medication. For example, he may feel that taking medication to relieve pain is a sign of weakness in a man. Following interventions such as these, some degree of compromise may be reached between nurse and patient, so that, for example, the latter may be prepared to take some small amount of medication immediately before physiotherapy but not at other times.

Evaluation

In formatively evaluating Riehl's model of nursing, attention is likely to focus on whether or not goals set at the planning stage have been achieved. This will usually involve an examination of the patient's behaviour to see to what extent he or she had been able to adopt new role performances or extend existing ones. It is important to realise, however, that nursing intervention can only be considered successful when the role performances which follow it enable patients to cope more effectively with pre-existing problems and the care itself.

Thus, when the mother-to-be is able to say that she is more confident in her ability to cope with her new baby, a significant goal will have been realised. Later on in formative evaluation, however, an attempt may be made to explore more fully the extent to which her expression of such attitudes has been accompanied by an increase in her ability to carry out effective child care.

Similarly, if following intervention the teenager is able to adopt the sick role to the extent where he is happy to receive some analgesia to enable nursing and other care to be carried out, then nursing intervention can be considered to have been effective.

Because formative evaluation is so closely linked to the re-assessment of patients' role-related needs in Riehl's model of nursing, those working with it are likely to undertake some assessment during each stage of the nursing process.

Summative evaluation will also prove essential with this model of nursing and is likely to focus particularly on the advantages and disadvantages of this model of care in meeting a variety of nursing needs.

9

Rogers's Unitary Field Model of Nursing

Introduction

In helping nurses to understand patients and their health-related needs, many of the models of nursing so far considered have focused either on the existence of physiological, psychological and social sub-systems within the individual or on the human quality of symbolising and 'making sense' of social experience. Some nurses, however, have argued that both of these rather different approaches to nursing practice share certain assumptions, since they take their origins from within what may be viewed as peculiarly *western* ways of understanding people and their needs.

In particular, the former approach, one that likens a person to a biological system with many parts, each with its own unique but inter-related function, shares many similarities with the dominant set of medical understandings which emerged in Western Europe following anatomical and physiological investigations in the seventeenth and eighteenth centuries. Such a set of understandings, it could be argued, by 'fragmenting' humans into parts, systems and sub-systems, each with their associated activities, suggests that people are best thought of as the sum of these structures and the functions for which they are responsible.

In a similar way, the interactionist perspective, which underpins models of nursing that emphasise people's abilities to symbolise and 'make sense' of their experience, also works with a peculiarly western way of seeing humans and their activities, since it views

85

people as rational individuals who piece together, from a fragmented world of experience, complex understandings about the self and its relationship to this world.

According to Blattner (1981), such perspectives about the nature of human beings, and, by extension, the nature of patients receiving nursing care, are quite different from more traditional ways of understanding people and their needs. In particular, they differ significantly from the understandings worked with by healers and health practitioners in the Asian subcontinent, the Americas and the Mediterranean world up to the sixteenth century.

The approaches to health care used in these contexts took exception to the belief that human beings and their functioning could be meaningfully fragmented in such a way. Instead they argued that people are best understood as *wholes*, rather than as the sum of their individual parts. Such an alternative perspective, that of *holism*, still influences the thinking of health practitioners in many parts of the world today, and the traditional medicines of both China and India still work to great effect from such a premise.

Krieger (1981), in analysing such holistic approaches to health care, has identified a number of recurrent themes among the health-related practices of North American Indian shamans, Chinese health-care experts and Indian Ayurvedic health practitioners, all of whom have traditionally worked with understandings of individuals and their needs which emphasise the impossibility of reducing the person to a set of parts or systems around which health practice might be focused. By identifying a number of recurrent concerns within such holistic approaches to health care, it should be possible to set the scene for a consideration of a model of nursing which works with such ideas: Rogers's Unitary Field model of nursing.

According to Eliade (1971), among many North American Indian societies it was, and to a lesser extent still is, widely believed that physical and psychological conditions as disparate as weakness, dizziness, feelings of confusion, fainting and many other health-related complaints are the result of problems associated with a fundamental source of energy in every person: the soul. Some of these problems may be caused by soul loss, some by the straying of the soul, yet others following the soul's possession by external forces. In such cases only the intervention of a Shaman (a person having special insight into the nature of such changes) could lead to the individual's return to a condition of relative normality. It is important to note, however, that the nature of intervention made by the Shaman was one directed towards the person as a whole, and to the presence or absence of the soul, rather than towards specific parts of the individual believed to require attention.

According to Krieger, similar emphases are also to be found in the work of Chinese healers from 500 BC onwards, many of whom believe that imbalances in the flow of energy within a person can lead to physical and psychological illness. According to the accounts they developed, life energy (Ch'i), which exists in many different forms, flows throughout the body in synarteries, its rate of flow being influenced by the relationship between the individual's body rhythms and those rhythms outside the person, in nature. Lunar and solar cycles, as well as metereological and climatic conditions, are believed to create systems of energy which interact with those within the person: the simultaneous, rhythmical interaction between energy fields within and outside the person being believed to determine a individual's state of well-being. Health-care interventions within such a framework again focus holistically upon the person, attempting to restore the free flow of life energy throughout the body and soul. Acupuncture, massage and moxybustion (applying the burning ash of the mugwort plant to sensitive points along synarteries), as well as the use of herbal remedies, are prime modes of intervention within such a holistic framework.

Similarly, Skeet (1978) argues that today, among Ayurvedic health practitioners on the Indian subcontinent, attention is directed towards holistically restoring the balance of three bodily humours—vata (wind), pitha (gall) and kapha (mucus)—within an ill person. Moreover, such practitioners believe that the harmonic interaction between these humours is something that can be easily thrown out of balance by a mismatch between person rhythms and those in nature. Ayurvedic health-care intervention, normally assessed as necessary following an examination of the quality of different pulses, is likely to involve the use of naturopathic remedies, changes in diet and physical activity, or forms of yoga to help re-establish the balance between the individual and the universe.

Finally, in the European holistic approach to health care used by the ancient Greeks and by followers of Galen after the second century, there exist similar emphases. The accounts offered by such writers identified the existence of four bodily humours: blood, mucus, yellow bile and black bile. Relative imbalance between these was said to result when individuals were out of balance with their environments. Within this tradition, diagnosis, once more carried out by means of an examination of bodily pulses, would be likely to be followed by health-care interventions to help re-establish harmony between the whole individual and the environment.

Throughout the above accounts run a number of important themes that have formed the basis for a more modern revival of interest in such approaches to health care. First, each of them emphasises *holism*, the belief that the entirety of the individual can never usefully be reduced to a consideration of its parts. Second, they each emphasise *rhythmicity*, the notion that there exist cycles and resonances between the physical and psychological functioning of humans and their environments. Finally, the theme of *potentiality* is present in each account: the idea that within people there exist untapped sources of energy which can be used for self-healing and the restoration of the person to a state of relative well-being.

Many of these ideas may sound unfamiliar and possibly even dangerous to nurses today. All the more so, perhaps, because contemporary patterns of nurse education often encourage an unquestioning acceptance of the idea that patients are best seen as sets of interrelated systems and functions. However, in the interests of an eclectic approach to nursing practice, it would seem unwise to reject all that more holistic approaches to care have to offer. In recent years, therefore, a number of nurses have begun to work with such ideas to develop more radical approaches to patient care.

Krieger, for example, has argued that the goal of modern holistic nursing care should be to '. . . treat all aspects of the person's problems by an integrated approach that considers both the person in the context of the problem and the problem in the context of the uniqueness of the individual, thus giving the situation a more humanistic orientation than has previously been the case . . .' In a wide-ranging survey of current approaches to holistic nursing practice, she cites with approval the increasing involvement of nurses in hypnotherapy, meditation and autogenic training as aids to patient relaxation, and in the use of biofeedback as a means of encouraging greater control over aspects of autonomic function. Furthermore, she advocates that nurses should become increasingly involved in chiropractice, aikido and dance therapy as means of facilitating a greater integrity between person and environment, and in the use of acupuncture, acupressure and therapeutic touch as a means of redistributing bodily energies.

The approach to nursing care that writers such as Krieger advocate is one that has been considerably influenced by the work of Rogers, who, for the past twenty years, has been working at New York University developing a holistic model of nursing. Since Rogers's (1970, 1980) work is, at present, probably the most fully developed holistic approach to nursing care, it would seem useful to explore how its commitments might be put into practice using the nursing process. As with other models, an attempt will be made first of all to examine what this particular model of nursing has to say about seven key aspects of people and patient care. Some suggestions will then be made about its possible use with the nursing process.

Key Components of Care

The Nature of People

According to Rogers, it is a mistake to view people as individuals functioning with physiological, psychological and social systems within them. Instead they should be viewed holistically. By doing this, nurses are likely to be able to begin to appreciate that those in their care are people who are much more than the sum of their individual parts.

For Rogers, humans are *unitary fields of energy* interacting with other energy fields in their vicinity. Human behaviours, arising out of such interactions between energy fields, should best be regarded holistically as what Rogers calls *synergistic processes*. According to such a view, nurses should not aim to make sense of particular behaviours in terms of their origins within a specific aspect of the person (be it an aspect related to a physiological, psychological or social sub-system). Instead they should recognise that behaviour arises from the *person as a whole* in interaction with the *environment as a whole*.

Through her work, Rogers claims to have identified three general principles about the nature of this interaction between energy systems.

The first principle, that of *complementarity*, argues that there is a constant interaction between the human energy field and environmental energy fields.

The second principle, that of *helicy*, is suggestive of the way in which human and environmental change takes place. Rogers believes, perhaps somewhat optimistically, that interaction between personal and environmental energy fields is such that continuous innovation and diversity of outcome is achieved. For her, both human and environmental development proceed from conditions of relative simplicity to greater complexity in a rhythmical manner. She uses the analogy of the well-known Slinky toy to suggest the nature of this development (Figure 9.1). Human and environmental energy fields change in both a directional (indicated by progression along the wire from one end of the Slinky to the other) and a rhythmical manner (indicated by the nature of the progression involved, recycling around the loops of the toy).

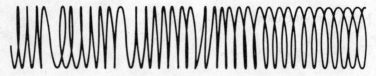

Figure 9.1   The Slinky toy

The third principle, that of *resonancy*, suggests that the interaction between human and environmental energy fields is patterned and ordered in its effects. In particular, Rogers argues that there is an evolutionary tendency for human behaviour to conform to higher patterns of frequency both within and across life cycles. As evidence supportive of this assertion, she identifies both hyperactivity in children and the more frequent patterns of sleeping and waking seen in the elderly as two examples of this general effect. However, unlike more pessimistic interpretations of these two types of behaviour, Rogers sees them as positive instances of human evolutionary development.

The Causes of Problems Likely to Require Nursing Intervention

According to Rogers's model of nursing, the major source of problems likely to require nursing intervention will be conditions of imbalance between human and environmental energy fields. Such a situation can result from three rather different sets of circumstances. First of all, a person might be overstimulated by environmental contingencies. Second, an individual might be understimulated by these same forces. Third, a condition of imbalance might arise from a mismatch between rhythmicities inherent in the individual and those in the immediate environment. Nursing intervention is likely to be required in any of these situations to assist the person to develop patterns of living that co-ordinate with, and match, the environmental energy field.

However, nursing intervention may, on some occasions, aim to achieve rather more than this, since it may be directed towards ensuring that the person avoids the likelihood of future conditions of imbalance. In this sense, Rogers's model of nursing anticipates that nurses may play a promotional role in health care.

The Nature of the Assessment Process

With many nursing models, assessment involves an examination of physiological, psychological and social aspects of the patient. According to Quinn (1981), however, nursing assessment using Rogers's holistic model of care should attempt to gain information about the organisation of the energy field within the person.

One of the most useful aids in performing this aspect of assessment is the use of therapeutic touch. Krieger (1979) has argued that, in using therapeutic touch to assess patients, nurses should move their hands over the body of the client, remaining sensitive to areas of heat and energy within. Naturally the acquisition of such a skill is something that must be learned in a rigorous and systematic way, and Krieger and her colleagues at New York University have worked actively to promote training programmes in the use of such a technique.

In addition to using this assessment technique, nurses should also attempt to receive as many other health-related signals from the client as possible. In aiming to achieve this, nurses may need to work actively to avoid a tendency to scan people and their attributes in a fragmented way. Rather efforts should be made to respond holistically to those in need of care. As Quinn puts it, in doing this, nurses are likely to use the energy fields of their own bodies to interact with those of patients by touching, holding and responding to them in a 'beautifully direct way'.

The Nature of the Planning and Goal-setting Process

Using this model of nursing, planning and goal-setting is likely to require the identification of a series of immediate and long-term goals. In the immediate sense, attention may need to be focused on problems causing what Rogers calls *dis-ease*. By this term Rogerian nurses mean to identify any immediate disturbances in the individual's energy field, not necessarily just those associated with the presence of pathogens. However, attention is also likely to be given to the setting of long-term goals, perhaps involving patients in a repatterning of their daily routines so that a more harmonious relationship between them and their environment can be developed.

The Focus of Intervention During the Implementation of the Care Plan

In a desire to use as broad an array of interventions as possible, nurses working with Rogers's model are unlikely to reject the use of drugs and technological innovations in their delivery of nursing care. Instead these may be used to help alleviate some of the more immediate causes of dis-ease. However, such nurses may well share some scepticism about the long-term value of such modes of intervention in the absence of concurrent attempts to rebalance energy within the person.

The use of therapeutic touch to 'unruffle the energy field' (Krieger, 1979), of the self in empathetic communication or of homoeopathic and naturopathic remedies will all fall within nurses' repertoire of available modes of intervention. The use of body massage, or rolfing (a form of deep body massage involving the movement of muscle blocks) or of acupuncture and acupressure may also prove to be useful adjuncts to nursing practice. At all times, however, the focus of nursing intervention during the delivery of care is likely to be on the whole person, and on the re-establishment of conditions of equilibrium between the patient's energy field and that of the immediate or potential environment.

The Nature of the Process of Evaluating the Quality and Effects of the Care Given

Quinn, in her writing exploring the use of Rogers's model of nursing with the nursing process, admits that evaluating the extent to which a nurse has been successful in repatterning the energy field within a person is unlikely to be a simple process. She suggests, however, that a number of different phenomena may be looked for which might indicate when nursing intervention has been relatively effective. First, the patient may show a greater awareness of the relationship between environmental factors and his or her problems. For example, following nursing intervention, individuals may show a greater awareness of the relationship between the work they do and their present health-related problems. More subtle changes, such as 'fullness where there was limpness' or 'balance where there was asymmetry', may take longer to discern, as may changes in the overall composure of patients and their energy fields.

The Role of the Nurse

According to Rogers (1970), the major concern of nursing is to '. . . promote symphonic interaction between man and environment, to strengthen the coherence and integrity of the human field, and to direct and re-direct patterning of the human and environmental fields for realisation of maximum health potential . . .'. Such a view would seem to suggest that the role of the nurse is primarily concerned with health and well-being. Indeed, Rogers suggests that nursing exists to serve people wherever they may be: at home, in school or in hospital. The uniqueness of every individual and the notion of potentiality implied by this model of nursing require that nurses should value people for themselves, while at the same time remaining aware of the limitations of some existing societal or medical norms. For example, Rogers's belief that evolutionary development can explain such phenomena as hypertension and hyperactivity, demands that nurses remain sensitive to the relativity of behavioural norms, This, in turn, may require nurses to develop imaginative methods of care in order to promote well-being.

Finally, given this model of nursing's concern with the interaction between human and environmental energy fields, nurses should remain aware that they constitute an environmental component for each person with whom they come into contact.

Using Rogers's Model of Nursing with the Nursing Process

The preceding outline of Rogers's model of nursing has tried to show that, no matter how unfamiliar ideas within it may seem for many nurses, there may nevertheless be value in the use of more holistic approaches to nursing care. By considering how the model might be used with the nursing process, some encouragement may be given to nurses who wish to evaluate its usefulness for the planning and delivery of care.

Assessment

For a Rogerian nurse it is imperative that the patient be viewed at all times as a coherent whole. Hence, assessment is likely to aim to gain information about the organisation of a person's overall energy field and about the relationship between this and that of the environment. Since Rogers stresses that changes are constantly occurring within this relationship, it would seem crucial that nurses involve themselves in a continuous process of assessment if their view of the patient is not to become too fragmented. Such an approach to assessment has also been advocated by Macrae (1981) in work developing more general approaches to holistic nursing assessment. Thus, for those working with Rogers's model of nursing, a two-stage assessment similar to that emphasised in some other models of nursing would not seem appropriate.

Assessment may use a number of techniques which help the nurse to remain alert to health-related signals. Such techniques are likely to include observation, conversation and therapeutic touch. Evidence from such health-related signals should then be integrated into an overall holistic assessment of the patient, to provide the nurse with information about the organisation of the person's energy field.

For example, a woman entering an accident and emergency department following an injury to her wrist might display a number

94

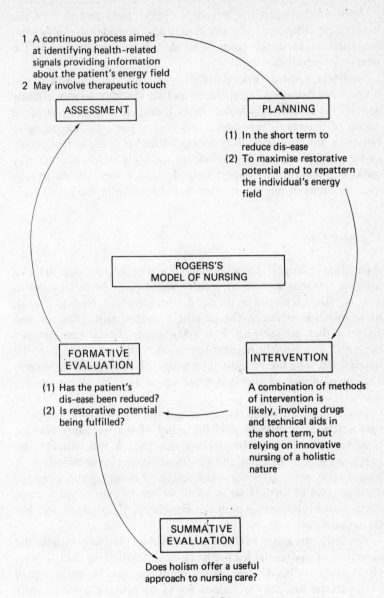

1 A continuous process aimed
at identifying health–related
signals providing information
about the patient's energy field
2 May involve therapeutic touch

ASSESSMENT

PLANNING

(1) In the short term to
reduce dis-ease
(2) To maximise restorative
potential and to repattern
the individual's energy
field

ROGERS'S
MODEL OF NURSING

FORMATIVE
EVALUATION

INTERVENTION

(1) Has the patient's
dis-ease been reduced?
(2) Is restorative potential
being fulfilled?

A combination of methods
of intervention is
likely, involving drugs
and technical aids in
the short term, but
relying on innovative
nursing of a holistic
nature

SUMMATIVE
EVALUATION

Does holism offer a useful
approach to nursing care?

Figure 9.2

of such health-related signals. Her avoidance of arm movements and her verbal expressions of anxiety may lead the nurse to identify a mismatch between the woman's energy field and that of the hospital environment. The nurse may also consider that a general overstimulation in the form of wrist pain is contributing to the woman's overall dis-ease.

Similarly, a nurse working in the community and visiting a man at home who describes leg stiffness and an inability to move easily around the house, may make use of therapeutic touch to become aware of the man's inner heat and energy pattern. According to Quinn, a 'normal' or healthy energy pattern is likely to feel evenly distributed, whereas differences from one body area to another may indicate a less healthy energy field. In such a way, the nurse may identify areas of energy imbalance and tension in the man's legs.

Planning Care

According to Rogers, the goal of nursing is to help patients to make a move towards a state of greater well-being. In this model of nursing, stress is placed on the need to set long-term goals as a result of negotiation between the patient and the nurse. Rogers also suggests that goal-setting, like assessment, should continuously evolve if a genuinely holistic approach to nursing care is to be maintained. The use of short-term goals, however, may be acceptable in planning to alleviate more immediate problems causing dis-ease.

In such ways the nurse in the accident and emergency department may set as a short-term goal the relief of the woman's dis-ease relating to her injury. In meeting this goal it will probably be necessary to use analgesia and a method of joint immobilisation. A longer-term goal, however, may relate to reducing the woman's present level of anxiety so as to allow her to experience a more harmonious relationship between her energy field and that of her immediate environment.

Similarly, the nurse in the community may plan to maximise the elderly man's potential for recovery by redistributing energy in an effort to relieve his dis-ease. An attempt may also be made to plan to repattern his daily activities so as to achieve greater unity between himself and the environment.

According to Rogers, nursing skill involves selecting the most appropriate means of intervention, so that the patient may be relieved of immediate dis-ease and can achieve a greater harmony with the environment. While accepting the use of traditional methods of care, Rogers suggests that, in order to respond holistically, the nurse may need to be imaginative and innovative in the application of nursing knowledge to practice.

For the woman in the accident and emergency department, it may be appropriate to both splint her wrist and offer analgesia in an effort to reduce the overstimulation to her energy field. At the same time, however, talking with and listening to her may enable the nurse to reduce the conflict between the woman's energy field and that of the hospital environment.

Intervention for the elderly man may involve the use of therapeutic touch by the nurse. According to Rogers, the use of therapeutic touch should take the form of a purposeful intervention aiming to help or heal. Thus, the nurse may use hand touch to transfer energy to her client in an effort to maximise his own restorative potential. An attempt may also be made to discuss with him ways in which his energy field may better match that of his environment.

Evaluation

Evaluating Rogers's model of nursing poses certain problems. As Quinn has pointed out, determining whether skin is broken or not can often be a relatively simple process, whereas making a judgement about the repatterning of a client's energy field is rather more complicated. Moreover, in her own writing, Rogers offers little guidance on evaluation. While a degree of formative evaluation may be possible to determine whether or not there has been an aimed-for reduction in dis-ease, nurses may have more difficulty in evaluating the appropriateness and relative success of particular nursing interventions in bringing about such changes. To some extent, such difficulties arise because this particular nursing model recommends the use of a wide range of novel interventions during the delivery of care.

This emphasises that evaluation, for nurses working with

Rogers's model of nursing, may at certain times be more straight-forward than at others. For example, it may be relatively simple to identify that a reduction in the woman's immediate dis-ease has taken place by asking her questions about this and by observing how pre-occupied she is with the pain in her wrist. It may be less easy, however, to establish whether her repatterned energy field will allow her now, and in the future, to enter a hospital environment with less anxiety.

Similarly, if the elderly man shows a greater awareness of those behaviours that help his energy field to harmonise more adequately with his environment (for example, he may avoid sitting still for long periods), and becomes more able to move around, the nurse may have some difficulty in linking the attainment of these particular goals to specific nursing interventions that have been made.

It would seem, therefore, that formative evaluation is likely to require both rigour and sensitivity from nurses seeking to evaluate the usefulness of Rogers's model of nursing.

In subjecting this holistic model of nursing to summative evalua-tion, nurses are likely to ask whether holism offers a useful approach to nursing care. In reaching decisions about this, not only will it be vital to evaluate the usefulness of Rogers's nursing model in a variety of nursing contexts, but also it will be necessary to explore the challenge which holism poses to more conventional approaches to patient care. Working with Rogers's model of nursing therefore may require nurses to justify their choice of an approach to care which may be perceived by others as being at odds with emphases shared by both the medical model and other models of nursing care.

10

From Nursing Models to Nursing Theory

Introduction

A number of models of nursing having been described and some suggestions having been made about how they may be put into practice with the nursing process, it would now seem appropriate to consider how nurses can choose between them. So far, in keeping with an intention to explore different models of care in a relatively open way, an attempt has been made to present the elements of each nursing model in as non-critical a manner as possible. Such an approach has deficiencies, however, since it may encourage some nurses to feel that it does not really matter which model of nursing is chosen to inform nursing practice in a particular care setting. It might further encourage the view that choosing between nursing models is something best done intuitively, as an act of personal preference. Even worse, it might encourage some nurses to feel that their everyday problems might be eliminated were they to make some sort of 'right choice' in selecting a particular model for use in a care setting or health district.

To take any of these courses of action would be to miss the main purpose underlying the development of conceptual models of nursing. As many of their originators have pointed out, nursing models are not to be seen as 'good' or 'bad', as 'right' or 'wrong'. Rather they should be used as *guidelines* within which to explore the appropriateness of particular approaches to care in different nursing contexts.

Evaluating Nursing Models

Deciding between nursing models is a task which needs to be undertaken with some degree of sensitivity, since choosing an inappropriate model with which to work may have undesirable consequences for both practising nurses and those in care. In the nursing literature, a number of writers have tried to identify criteria which can help nurses to make decisions about which nursing model to use. It would seem useful, therefore, to identify a number of different suggestions that have been made, before attempting to identify some of the features they have in common.

One of the first frameworks by which different nursing models could be contrasted was that suggested by Riehl and Roy (1980). They argued that conceptual models of nursing could be compared in terms of what they have to say about the eight aspects of nursing and patient care identified in Table 10.1. More recent writers, however, have argued that a number of qualitatively different steps are involved in the critical evaluation of different nursing models. Chinn and Jacobs (1983), for example, while failing to differentiate as clearly as might have been done between nursing models and nursing theories, argue that there exists a distinction between *describing* and *evaluating* nursing models.

Table 10.1 Framework for comparison of nursing models (Riehl and Roy, 1980)

---

(1) *Assumptions* made about people and their behaviour
(2) *Values* held about the role of nursing in patient care
(3) The *goal* of nursing as a profession
(4) The nature of who or what is acted upon in achieving nursing goals (the whole person, a system within them, etc.). Riehl and Roy call this *patiency*
(5) The *role of the nurse* in achieving goals
(6) The *source of difficulty* believed to give rise to problems needing nursing intervention
(7) The *focus* and *mode* of *interventions* made by the nurse
(8) The *intended* and *unintended consequences* likely to result from nursing interventions

---

In describing a model, nurses are likely to identify *goals* it presupposes for nursing, *concepts* from which it is built, *relationships* between these which it argues for and *assumptions* which it works with. Additionally, interest is likely to be shown in its *power* and *breadth* with respect to the range of nursing activities about which it has something to say. This range of activities is similar to that earlier identified by Riehl and Roy.

In evaluating a nursing model, however, Chinn and Jacobs argue that the qualities identified in Table 10.2 should be looked at. In exploring how lucid a model is, attention should be directed towards both the *clarity* with which concepts are defined and used (this is what Chinn and Jacobs call the semantic and structural clarity of a model) and the *consistency* with which such concepts are employed (this they describe as a model's semantic and structural consistency). In evaluating a model's *simplicity*, nurses should look for the minimum number of concepts and relationships within it. A model with *generality* can explain a wide range of phenomena of interest to nurses. Finally, in exploring what Chinn and Jacobs call a model's *empirical precision* and the *derivable consequences* which follow from this, nurses should turn their attention to how well the model can predict what actually happens in the real world of nursing.

This distinction between descriptive and evaluative criteria used in comparing nursing models is a useful one, but is one that has been further refined in recent years.

Fawcett (1980, 1984), for example, has also distinguished between description and evaluation in her comparison of different models of nursing (in fact, she calls the process of description

Table 10.2   Aspects involved in evaluating nursing theory/models
(Chinn and Jacobs, 1983)

---

(1) Exploring their *semantic and structural clarity*
(2) Exploring their *semantic and structural consistency*
(3) Looking at their *simplicity*
(4) Looking at their *generality*
(5) Looking at their *empirical precision*
(6) Looking at their ability to *predict* derivable consequences

---

analysis). She argues that, during each of these processes, attention should be focused on the issues identified in Tables 10.3 and 10.4.

Table 10.3 Issues that should receive attention in analysing (describing) nursing models (Fawcett, 1984)

(1) The way in which a model has been *developed*
(2) The *concepts* and *propositions* that the model works with. In particular, what it has to say about:
    (a) how *people* are defined and described
    (b) how the *environment* is defined and described
    (c) how *health* is defined and described
    (d) how *nursing* and its goals are defined and described
(3) What *areas of nursing concern* the model focuses on

Table 10.4 Issues that should receive attention in evaluating nursing models (Fawcett, 1984)

(1) How well identified its *assumptions* are
(2) How *comprehensive* its concepts and propositions are
(3) The *logical congruence* or degree of fit between its various propositions and assumptions
(4) The *social considerations* it works with. In particular, the relationship which it advocates nurses should have with the wider society
(5) Its ability either to *generate* or *test* nursing theory
(6) The value of the contribution it offers to *nursing knowledge*

Similar themes are to be found in the writing of Meleis (1985), who argues that an analysis of nursing models should be followed by a systematic critique.

In analysing a model of nursing, Meleis argues, attention should be paid to three main areas of concern: the *theorist*, the *paradigmatic origins* of the model and its *internal dimensions*. While a more complete description of what is meant by each of these terms is to be found in Meleis' own writing, in enquiring into aspects of the theorist, the nurse should aim to ask questions about the educational and professional background of the model's originator, as well as about the culture in which she or he works. In exploring the paradigmatic origins of a nursing model, Meleis advocates that nurses should aim to identify the origins of assumptions with which a model works, key concepts and relationships within it, and nursing hypotheses to which it gives rise. Finally, in looking at the internal dimensions of a model, nurses might aim to explore its scope, the range of nursing applications it aims to influence, the propositions it makes about nursing, the goals that it sees for nursing, its degree of abstractness and the methods which have been used to develop it.

Such a process of *analysis* is likely to go well beyond the level of description argued for by writers such as Riehl and Roy or Chinn and Jacobs. However, it may not go far enough in terms of enabling an effective and critical evaluation of different nursing models to take place. To achieve this, Meleis advocates a further exploration of the following four aspects of nursing models, in a process which she describes as *critique* (Table 10.5).

In looking at the relationship between *structure* and *function* implied by a nursing model, Meleis believes, it is important to look at how clearly concepts within it are articulated. Do they overlap with one another in any way? Are the relationships between them clearly specified? Is there needless repetition within the account of the model? Are the ideas it puts forward either too complex or too simple for the issues that it addresses?

Table 10.5　Aspects of a nursing model to be explored when subjecting it to critique (Meleis, 1985)

---

(1) Is the model clear in *structure and function*?
(2) What has been the model's *circle of contagiousness*?
(3) What is the model's potential *usefulness* for:
    (a) nursing practice?
    (b) nursing research?
    (c) nurse education?
    (d) nursing administration?
(4) What relationships exist between the nursing values espoused by a model and
    (a) the values of other health professions?
    (b) dominant beliefs and expectations in society?

In exploring what she calls the *circle of contagiousness* of a model, Meleis directs attention to whether or not a model has been taken up and used by others. She notes that some models of nursing have spread widely across institutions, whereas others have not. She argues that nursing models whose use has spread geographically from their place of origin are likely to be those found most useful by practising nurses.

In encouraging an exploration of the *usefulness* of nursing models, Meleis invites reflection on their practical significance. Some may facilitate innovation in nursing practice, others in nurse education, yet others in systems of nurse management. Nursing models with breadth and power may be able to produce change in all three of these aspects of nursing, although, in evaluating a particular model, care should be taken to remember the scope that its originator intended it to have.

Finally, by advocating an examination of the relationship between values implicit in a model of nursing and those shared by other health-care professionals and society at large, Meleis encourages an exploration of the external relations true of a particular nursing model. By doing this, she signals that conceptual models of nursing can not be evaluated in isolation from the broader social and institutional context in which they are used.

The preceding ways of analysing and evaluating nursing models have identified a number of important criteria for nurses to bear in mind when deciding which one to work with. However, as will be apparent, nurse theorists disagree with one another in terms of the issues which they consider it important to explore in comparing models of nursing. It would seem useful, therefore, to present a simplified set of questions that might be asked about any model before considering its use in nursing practice. The following list does not claim to be exhaustive, but identifies a number of critical questions nurses might ask in deciding between different conceptual models of nursing.

(1) What *assumptions* does a model make about people and their health-related needs? How well do these assumptions match the nurse's understanding of people and their health-related needs?

(2) What *values* does a model work with?

(3) What are the key *concepts* a model uses? Are these useful in making sense of nursing and caring for people? Have they been

derived from work in other disciplines, or have they emerged from the research and concerns of professional nurses?

(4) What *relationships* are suggested between these concepts? Do these seem reasonable in the light of nursing experience? Is there nursing research to support the existence of these relationships?

(5) How does the model see the *role* of the nurse? Is this conception of role recognised and accepted by practising nurses?

(6) Is the model *parsimonious* and to the point, and yet not too simplistic?

(7) Does the model have something of *generality* to say about nursing in the context in which its use is being considered?

(8) Is the use of the model likely to lead to better *standards of care*?

By asking questions such as these, practising nurses, nurse managers and nurse educators may be able to make more informed judgements about the relative strengths of different nursing models in meeting particular needs. However, deciding which model to work with in a particular nursing context is only the first step in a process of critical enquiry, since, after a model has been selected and used, nurses are likely to want to explore how well it lived up to their expectations. In reaching a decision about this, and in completing the process of evaluation, a further set of questions is likely to be asked. Again it is difficult to provide a definitive list, but the following are among those most likely to be asked.

(1) Did the nursing model provide guidelines on assessment which enabled the patient's problems to be clearly identified?

(2) Did the planning of care and the setting of goals match the patient's expectations for care?

(3) Did the model suggest a range of nursing interventions that were practical in that particular care setting?

(4) Did the nursing interventions carried out enable the nurse to provide a standard of care acceptable to her/himself and the patient?

By subjecting conceptual models of nursing to a process of critical evaluation such as this, it should be possible to refine and develop them. Certain of their propositions may thereby come to be clarified and others rejected. Moreover, the types of nursing for which particular models are suitable may further come to be better understood. In such ways a move may be made towards the development of rather more definitive *nursing theories*. In the final section of this chapter an attempt will be made to identify some of the ways in which the development of nursing theory might take place.

Developing Nursing Theory

In recent years a number of writers have taken care to distinguish conceptual models of nursing from nursing theories. Chinn and Jacobs (1983), for example, have argued that '. . . Conceptual models may form preliminary or competing structures that will, with application of rigorous methods, evolve into (. . .) theory . . .'. Similarly, Fawcett (1984) has claimed that '. . . The primary distinction between a conceptual model and a theory is the level of abstraction. A conceptual model is a highly abstract system of global concepts and linking statements. A theory, in contrast, deals with one or more specific, concrete concepts and propositions . . .'. Moreover, both Chinn and Jacobs (1983) and Thibodeau (1983) have argued that developed nursing theories are likely to be predictive in the statements they make about effective nursing.

Taken together, such statements suggest, first of all, that nursing theories are likely to take their origins from conceptual models of nursing. Second, they suggest that, whereas conceptual models of nursing are often relatively abstract, nursing theories are more concrete and specific, perhaps dealing with a more limited number of events and situations. It may be useful, therefore, to think of nursing theories as strong nursing models, ones that have been tried and tested in a variety of nursing situations. Saying this, however, does not identify with any precision the process by which either nursing models or nursing theories come to be developed. In order to appreciate the nature of this process more fully, it seems useful to explore some of the general strategies that exist for theory development.

Broadly speaking, there are two main ways in which nursing models and theories can develop. The first of these begins with observations made by nurses in their everyday work. For example, if it is noticed that patients receiving one form of nursing care recover more quickly than those receiving an alternative style, it might be concluded that the former approach is in some sense superior to the latter. Such a strategy for theory development, in which a move is made from specific observations to general explanations, is sometimes called an *inductive* approach.

Alternatively, the starting point for the development of nursing models and theories can be ideas already present in existing natural, medical or social science theory. For example, social psychologists have known for some time that stress levels in people can be altered by the knowledge they have about the situations in which they find themselves. Taking such insights as a starting point, it might be possible to derive a series of hypotheses (tentative ideas) that can be tested in nursing practice. For example, it might be suggested that giving patients fuller information about the clinical and nursing procedures they are to undergo reduces the amount of stress experienced. Such an approach to theory development, in which existing research findings are used as the starting point for the identification of new nursing hypotheses to be tested, is a *hypothetico-deductive* approach to model and theory development.

More recently a third strategy for the development of nursing models and theories has been identified. Fawcett (1984) has described this as a *retroductive* strategy, one that combines aspects of both inductive and hypothetico-deductive approaches. Here the starting point is a series of observations thought to be related to one another. By detecting regularities among these, the nurse aims to identify a series of nursing concepts that help to 'make sense' of the relationships between them. Finally, the validity of such concepts and the relationships hypothesised to exist between them can be tested by nurses in situations other than those in which they were originally induced.

It is questionable, however, whether identifying nursing concepts and relationships between them can ever be a process entirely uninfluenced by existing theory. After all, how do nurses know which aspects of a patient's behaviour to focus on, unless their perceptions are influenced by theories about the significance (or otherwise) of certain behaviour? In recognising such a problem, Meleis (1985) has advocated the pursuit of what she has called a theory–research–theory strategy for the development of nursing knowledge. This begins by recognising that nurses must work with some sort of theory 'making sense' of events around them. Some of these theoretical frameworks may derive from models of care with which the nurse is familiar. Others may have their origin in natural and social scientific understandings with which the nurse is acquainted. Nevertheless, both of these different types of framework can generate ideas to be tested out in nursing practice. The outcome of this can be a refining of nursing models and, ultimately, the development of nursing theory.

More recently it has been argued that, by using the nursing process in conjunction with a model of nursing, nurses can combine both inductive and hypothetico-deductive commitments in critically evaluating nursing models and generating nursing theory. In particular, Aggleton and Chalmers (1986) have argued that, by systematically assessing patients using a nursing model, nurses can detect regularities among the observations made: patterns which may be the beginnings of inductively generated theoretical insights. By subsequently planning care in the light of these insights, and by implementing this according to a clearly defined plan, it may be possible to begin to test such newly developed nursing theory. Furthermore, by evaluating the extent to which intervention has been successful in meeting goals identified during the planning of care, nurses can further develop the inductively generated ideas about nursing that underpinned the approach to care used.

. . . In much the same way that systematic patient assessment carried out using a nursing model can create the possibility of inductively generating nursing theory, a careful evaluation of the outcomes of nursing interventions can allow a preliminary testing of this to take place . . . (Aggleton and Chalmers, 1986).

It may, therefore, be possible to combine both inductive and hypothetico-deductive commitments to theory development by using the nursing process to plan and deliver care around a chosen nursing model.

In this book we have tried to identify a number of ways in which nursing theory and nursing practice can be brought closer together. We have argued that one way in which this might take place would be for practising nurses to make fuller use of conceptual models of nursing as guidelines for their everyday nursing practice. We advocate this, not because we believe that practical nursing should be theory-led, but because we believe that a critical evaluation of different models of care requires that their claims be tested against the realities of everyday nursing practice. We see the bringing together of theory and practice in this way as a powerful and creative impetus for the production of nursing knowledge and for nursing's development as an autonomous set of theoretically informed health-care practices. If nurses reading this book feel inspired to accept the challenges and opportunities likely to be found in working with nursing models, our aims will have been achieved. If the outcome of this is a refinement of existing conceptual frameworks so that standards of nursing care are improved, then our hopes will have been more than realised.

References

Abbey, J. (1980). 'FANCAP: What is it?'. In J. P. Riehl and C. Roy (Eds.), *Conceptual Models for Nursing Practice* (Norwalk: Appleton-Century-Crofts)

Adam, E. (1980). *To Be a Nurse* (Eastbourne: Saunders)

Aggleton, P. J. and Chalmers, H. A. (1986). 'Nursing research, nursing theory and the nursing process', *Journal of Advanced Nursing*, **11**

Bandura, A. (1969). *Principles of Behaviour Modification* (New York: Harper and Row)

Black, N., Boswell, D., Gray, A., Murphy, S. and Popay, J. (Eds.) (1984). *Health and Disease: A Reader* (Milton Keynes: Open University Press)

Blattner, B. (1981). *Holistic Nursing* (Englewood Cliffs, N. J.: Prentice-Hall)

Bonney, V. and Rothberg, J. (1963). *Nursing Diagnosis and Therapy—An Instrument for Evaluation and Measurement* (New York: The League Exchange, National League for Nursing)

Burton, M. (1985). 'The Environment, good interactions and interpersonal skills in nursing'. In Kagan, C. (Ed.), *Interpersonal Skills in Nursing* (London: Croom Helm)

Butterfield, S. E. (1983). 'In search of commonalities: An analysis of two theoretical frameworks', *International Journal of Nursing Studies*, **20**, 15–22

Chinn, P. L. and Jacobs, M. K. (1983). *Theory and Nursing* (St. Louis: Mosby)

Coutu, W. (1951). 'Role-playing versus role-taking: An appeal for clarification', *American Sociological Review*, **16**, 180–187

Crow, J. (1977). 'The nursing process: 1', *Nursing Times*, **73**, 892–896

Duldt, B. W. and Giffin, K. (1985). *Theoretical Perspectives for Nursing* (Boston: Little Brown)

Eliade, M. (1971). *Shamanism* (Princeton, N. J.: Princeton University Press)

Faulkner, A. (1985). 'The organisational context of interpersonal skills in nursing'. In Kagan, C. (Ed.), *Interpersonal Skills in Nursing* (London: Croom Helm)

Fawcett, J. (1978). 'The relationship between theory and research: A double helix', *Advances in Nursing Science*, **1** (1), 49–62

Fawcett, J. (1980). 'A framework for analysis and evaluation of conceptual models of nursing', *Nurse Educator*, **5** (6), 10–14

Fawcett, J. (1984). *Analysis and Evaluation of Conceptual Models of Nursing* (Philadelphia: F. A. Davis)

Fitzpatrick, J. J. and Whall, A. L. (1983). *Conceptual Models of Nursing: Analysis and Application* (Bowie, Maryland: Robert J. Brady)

Fitzpatrick, R. M. (1983). 'Social concepts of disease and illness'. In Patrick, D. L. and Scambler, G. (Eds.), *Sociology as Applied to Medicine* (London: Baillière Tindall)

Grubbs, J. (1980). 'The Johnson Behavioural System Model'. In Riehl, J. P. and Roy, C. (Eds.), *Conceptual Models for Nursing Practice* Norwalk: Appleton-Century-Crofts)

Hall, C. (1983). 'A time for reflection', *Journal of Advanced Nursing*, **8**, 457–466

Henderson, V. (1966). *The Nature of Nursing: A Definition and its Implications for Practice, Research and Education* (New York: Macmillan)

Henderson, V. (1972). *Basic Principles of Nursing Care* (Geneva: International Council of Nurses)

Helson, H. (1964). *Adaptation Level Theory* (New York: Harper and Row)

Hull, C. L. (1951). *Essentials of Behaviour* (New Haven, Conn.: Yale University Press)

Illich, I. (1976). *Limits to Medicine* (Harmondsworth: Penguin)

Johnson, D. (1980). 'The Behavioural System Model for nursing'. In Riehl, J. P. and Roy, C. (Eds.), *Conceptual Models for Nursing Practice* (Norwalk: Appleton-Century-Crofts)

Kennedy, I. (1983). *The Unmasking of Medicine* (London: Granada)

Kratz, C. (1979). *The Nursing Process* (London: Baillière Tindall)

Krieger, D. (1979). *Therapeutic Touch: How to Use Your Hands to Help or Heal* (Englewood Cliffs, N. J.: Prentice-Hall)

Krieger, D. (Ed.) (1981). *Foundations for Holistic Health Nursing Practices* (Philadelphia: Lippincott)

Little, D. E. and Carnevali, D. L. (1971). 'The nursing care planning system', *Nursing Outlook*, **19**, 164–167

Macrae, J. A. (1981). 'Listening: An essay on the nature of holistic assessment'. In Krieger, D. (Ed.), *Foundations for Holistic Health Nursing Practices* (Philadelphia: Lippincott)

Marriner, A. (1979). *The Nursing Process* (St. Louis: Mosby)

Maslow, A. (1970). *Motivation and Personality* (New York: Harper and Row)

Mayers, M. C. (1972). *A Systematic Approach to the Nursing Care Plan* (New York: Appleton-Century-Crofts)

Mead, G. H. (1934). *Mind, Self and Society* (Chicago: University of Chicago Press)

Meleis, A. I. (1985). *Theoretical Nursing: Development and Progress* (Philadelphia: Lippincott)

Miller, A. (1985). 'The relationship between nursing theory and nursing practice', *Journal of Advanced Nursing*, **10**, 417–424

Orem, D. (1980). *Nursing: Concepts of Practice*, 2nd edn. (New York: McGraw-Hill)

Orem, D. (1985). *Nursing: Concepts of Practice*, 3rd edn. (New York: McGraw-Hill)

Quinn, J. F. (1981). 'Client care and nurse involvement in a holistic framework'. In Krieger, D. (Ed.), *Foundations For Holistic Health Nursing Practices* (Philadelphia: Lippincott)

Reynolds, B. (1985). 'Issues arising from teaching interpersonal skills in psychiatric nurse training'. In Kagan, C. (Ed.), *Interpersonal Skills in Nursing* (London: Croom Helm)

Riehl, J. P. (1980). 'The Riehl Interaction Model'. In Riehl, J. P. and Roy, C. (Eds.), *Conceptual Models for Nursing Practice* (Norwalk: Appleton-Century-Crofts)

Riehl, J. P. (1985). Personal communication

Riehl, J. P. and Roy, C. (Eds.) (1980). *Conceptual Models for Nursing Practice* (Norwalk: Appleton-Century-Crofts)

Rogers, C. (1951). *Client-Centred Therapy* (Boston: Houghton Mifflin)

Rogers, M. E. (1970). *An Introduction to the Theoretical Basis of Nursing* (Philadelphia: F. A. Davis)

Rogers, M. E. (1980). 'Nursing: A science of unitary man'. In Riehl, J. P. and Roy, L. C. (Eds.), *Conceptual Models for Nursing Practice* (Norwalk: Appleton-Century-Crofts)

Roper, N. (1976). *Clinical Experience in Nurse Education* (Edinburgh: Churchill Livingstone)

Roper, N., Logan, W. W. and Tierney, A. J. (1980). *The Elements of Nursing* (Edinburgh: Churchill Livingstone)

Roper, N., Logan, W. W. and Tierney, A. J. (1981). *Learning to Use the Process of Nursing* (Edinburgh: Churchill Livingstone)

Roper, N., Logan, W. W. and Tierney, A. J. (1983). *Using A Model for Nursing* (Edinburgh: Churchill Livingstone)

Roy, C. (1980). 'The Roy Adaptation Model'. In Riehl, J. P. and Roy, C. (Eds.), *Conceptual Models for Nursing Practice* (Norwalk: Appleton-Century-Crofts)

Roy, C. (1984). *Introduction to Nursing: An Adaptation Model* (Englewood Cliffs, N. J.: Prentice-Hall)

Roy, C. and Roberts, S. (1981). *Theory Construction in Nursing: An Adaptation Model* (Englewood Cliffs, N. J.: Prentice-Hall)

Skeet, M. (1978). 'Health auxiliaries: Decision-makers and implementers'. In Skeet, M. and Elliot, K. (Eds.) *Health Auxiliaries and the Health Team* (London: Croom Helm)

Thibodeau, J. A. (1983). *Nursing Models: Analysis and Evaluation* (Monterey, California: Wadsworth Health Sciences Division)

Thomas, W. I. (1967). *The Unadjusted Girl* (New York: Harper and Row)

Travelbee, J. (1966). *Interpersonal Aspects of Nursing* (Philadelphia: F. A. Davis)

Wiedenbach, E. (1964). *Clinical Nursing: A Helping Art* (New York: Springer Verlag)

Yura, H. and Walsh, M. B. (1967). *The Nursing Process* (Norwalk: Appleton-Century-Crofts)

Index